Emergency Medicine Evidence

The Practice-Changing Studies

Emily L. Aaronson, MD
Chief Resident
Harvard Affiliated Emergency
   Medicine Residency
Department of Emergency
   Medicine
Brigham and Women's Hospital
Massachusetts General Hospital
Boston, Massachusetts

Erik L. Antonsen, MD, PhD
Assistant Professor of Medicine
Section of Emergency Medicine
Assistant Professor of Space
   Medicine
Center for Space Medicine
Baylor College of Medicine
Attending Physician
Ben Taub General Hospital
Houston, Texas

Arjun K. Venkatesh, MD, MBA, MHS
Director, Quality and Safety Research
   and Strategy
Instructor, Department of Emergency
   Medicine
Scientist, Center for Outcomes
   Research and Evaluation
Yale University School of Medicine
New Haven, Connecticut

SPECIAL EDITORS

Ron M. Walls, MD, FACEP, FRCPC
Jonathan N. Adler, MD, MS, FACEP, FAAEM

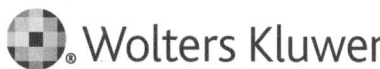

Philadelphia • Baltimore • New York • London
Buenos Aires • Hong Kong • Sydney • Tokyo

Acquisitions Editor: Jamie M. Elfrank
Product Development Editor: Ashley Fischer
Production Product Manager: David Saltzberg
Senior Manufacturing Manager: Beth Welsh
Marketing Manager: Stephanie Manzo
Design Coordinator: Teresa Mallon
Production Service: Aptara, Inc.

© 2015 by Wolters Kluwer Health
Two Commerce Square
2001 Market Street
Philadelphia, Pa. 19103 USA
LWW.com

All rights reserved. This book is protected by copyright. No part of this book may be reproduced in any form by any means, including photocopying, or utilized by any information storage and retrieval system without written permission from the copyright owner, except for brief quotations embodied in critical articles and reviews. Materials appearing in this book prepared by individuals as part of their official duties as U.S. government employees are not covered by the above-mentioned copyright.

Printed in China

Library of Congress Cataloging-in-Publication Data
Available upon request

ISBN 978-1-4511-9298-8

Care has been taken to confirm the accuracy of the information presented and to describe generally accepted practices. However, the authors, editors, and publisher are not responsible for errors or omissions or for any consequences from application of the information in this book and make no warranty, expressed or implied, with respect to the currency, completeness, or accuracy of the contents of the publication. Application of the information in a particular situation remains the professional responsibility of the practitioner.

The authors, editors, and publisher have exerted every effort to ensure that drug selection and dosage set forth in this text are in accordance with current recommendations and practice at the time of publication. However, in view of ongoing research, changes in government regulations, and the constant flow of information relating to drug therapy and drug reactions, the reader is urged to check the package insert for each drug for any change in indications and dosage and for added warnings and precautions. This is particularly important when the recommended agent is a new or infrequently employed drug.

Some drugs and medical devices presented in the publication have Food and Drug Administration (FDA) clearance for limited use in restricted research settings. It is the responsibility of the health care provider to ascertain the FDA status of each drug or device planned for use in their clinical practice.

To purchase additional copies of this book, call our customer service department at (800) 638-3030 or fax orders to (301) 223-2320. International customers should call (301) 223-2300.

Visit Lippincott Williams & Wilkins on the Internet: at LWW.com. Lippincott Williams & Wilkins customer service representatives are available from 8:30 am to 6 pm, EST.

10 9 8 7 6 5 4 3 2 1

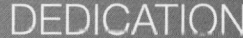

DEDICATION

I dedicate this book to my friends and family, who have all helped pave this way.
Emily L. Aaronson, MD

I dedicate this book to my parents, Larry and Pat Antonsen.
Erik L. Antonsen, MD, PhD

I dedicate this book to my wife Pooja Agrawal.
Arjun K. Venkatesh, MD, MBA, MHS

CONTRIBUTORS

Ije Akunyili, MD, MPA
Assistant Professor of Medicine
Section of Emergency Medicine
Baylor College of Medicine
Staff Emergency Physician
Memorial Hermann Southwest Hospital
Houston, Texas

Kenneth Bernard, MD
Resident Physician
Harvard Affiliated Emergency Medicine Residency
Department of Emergency Medicine
Brigham and Women's Hospital
Massachusetts General Hospital
Boston, Massachusetts

David Beversluis, MD, MPH
Resident Physician
Harvard Affiliated Emergency Medicine Residency
Department of Emergency Medicine
Brigham and Women's Hospital
Massachusetts General Hospital
Boston, Massachusetts

Michael E. Billington, MD
Resident Physician
Harvard Affiliated Emergency Medicine Residency
Department of Emergency Medicine
Brigham and Women's Hospital
Massachusetts General Hospital
Boston, Massachusetts

Stephanie E. Burgos, MD
Resident Physician
Harvard Affiliated Emergency Medicine Residency
Department of Emergency Medicine
Brigham and Women's Hospital
Massachusetts General Hospital
Boston, Massachusetts

Jennifer Carnell, MD
Assistant Professor of Medicine
Director of Emergency Ultrasound
Section of Emergency Medicine
Baylor College of Medicine
Houston, Texas

Brock Daniels, MD, MPH
Clinical Instructor
Department of Emergency Medicine
Yale-New Haven Hospital
Yale University School of Medicine
New Haven, Connecticut

Andrew J. Eyre, MD
Resident Physician
Harvard Affiliated Emergency Medicine Residency
Department of Emergency Medicine
Brigham and Women's Hospital
Massachusetts General Hospital
Boston, Massachusetts

Silpa Gadiraju, MD
Assistant Professor of Medicine
Section of Emergency Medicine
Baylor College of Medicine
Houston, Texas

Harman S. Gill, MD
Critical Care Medicine Fellow
Cleveland Clinic
Cleveland, Ohio

Spencer Greene, MD, MS, FACEP
Assistant Professor of Medicine
Director of Medical Toxicology
Section of Emergency Medicine
Baylor College of Medicine
Houston, Texas

Contributors

Kathryn Hawk, MD
Clinical Instructor
Drug Abuse, Addiction and HIV Research Scholar
Department of Emergency Medicine
Yale-New Haven Hospital
Yale University School of Medicine
New Haven, Connecticut

Eva Tovar Hirashima, MD
Resident Physician
Harvard Affiliated Emergency Medicine Residency
Department of Emergency Medicine
Brigham and Women's Hospital
Massachusetts General Hospital
Boston, Massachusetts

Joshua M. Keegan, MD
Resident Physician
Emergency Medicine Residency
Department of Emergency Medicine
Yale-New Haven Hospital
Yale University School of Medicine
New Haven, Connecticut

Ashley R. Kochanek, MD
Resident Physician
Harvard Affiliated Emergency Medicine Residency
Department of Emergency Medicine
Brigham and Women's Hospital
Massachusetts General Hospital
Boston, Massachusetts

Kito Lord, MD
Chief Resident
Emergency Medicine Residency
Department of Emergency Medicine
Yale-New Haven Hospital
Yale University School of Medicine
New Haven, Connecticut

Daphne Morrison Ponce, MD
Chief Resident
Harvard Affiliated Emergency Medicine Residency
Department of Emergency Medicine
Brigham and Women's Hospital
Massachusetts General Hospital
Boston, Massachusetts

Sabrina J. Poon, MD
Resident Physician
Harvard Affiliated Emergency Medicine Residency
Department of Emergency Medicine
Brigham and Women's Hospital
Massachusetts General Hospital
Boston, Massachusetts

Peter B. Pruitt, MD
Resident Physician
Harvard Affiliated Emergency Medicine Residency
Department of Emergency Medicine
Brigham and Women's Hospital
Massachusetts General Hospital
Boston, Massachusetts

Anita Rohra, MD
Assistant Professor of Medicine
Section of Emergency Medicine
Baylor College of Medicine
Houston, Texas

Paulina B. Sergot, MD
Assistant Professor of Medicine
Section of Emergency Medicine
Baylor College of Medicine
Houston, Texas

Radhika Sundararajan, MD, PhD
Resident Physician
Harvard Affiliated Emergency Medicine Residency
Department of Emergency Medicine
Brigham and Women's Hospital
Massachusetts General Hospital
Boston, Massachusetts

Christina Wilson, MD
Resident Physician
Harvard Affiliated Emergency Medicine Residency
Department of Emergency Medicine
Brigham and Women's Hospital
Massachusetts General Hospital
Boston, Massachusetts

David Yamane, MD
Resident Physician
Harvard Affiliated Emergency Medicine Residency
Department of Emergency Medicine
Brigham and Women's Hospital
Massachusetts General Hospital
Boston, Massachusetts

Fan Yang, MD
Resident Physician
Harvard Affiliated Emergency Medicine Residency
Department of Emergency Medicine
Brigham and Women's Hospital
Massachusetts General Hospital
Boston, Massachusetts

PREFACE

Why do we order the tests and treatments for our patients in the emergency department every shift? Over the past 20 years, evidence-based medicine has not only become an accepted lexicon in the practice of emergency medicine, but it has also elevated the standard of care for patients with acute, unscheduled illness across the nation. Evidence provides direction for our current interventions and creates future pathways for research to improve emergency care. Without clinical evidence we can neither make recommendations to our patients nor be sure we are providing the best available care.

When we were in medical school and later in residency, we often found ourselves challenged by attendings and senior residents to provide evidence to support our medical decision making. Often, they would quote a paper or a landmark clinical trial that we had not yet encountered. The first time someone refers to the "Rivers Trial" for sepsis, students and residents often are left wondering what it is or why it was important. Learners go through a painful process of searching through studies, being educated piecemeal by peers and looking for resources that put these studies into the appropriate historical and clinical context. Amidst the hundreds of topics that we seek to master, the challenge of identifying which studies were truly important to current practice, reading and interpreting them can seem insurmountable. Most importantly, identifying how we can apply the complex statistics and the findings to the clinical environment that we are practicing in is often challenging. This book seeks to provide the context for current clinical practice by discussing the most practice-changing original research studies that affected emergency medicine.

While the evolution of evidence-based medicine has improved health outcomes for numerous illnesses that present to the emergency department every day, several new challenges have emerged. First, the recommendation made in nearly 40% of research studies used to support medical practices may be reversed within a decade, suggesting that little clinical evidence stands the test of time. Second, despite compelling results in multiple research studies, clinicians still fail to follow evidence-based recommendations almost half the time. Our hope is that this book will help pick out those studies that have been most influential in advancing the quality of emergency care, while framing them in a way accessible to students, residents and practicing emergency physicians taking care of patients every day.

This book is a compilation of the 100 *most practice-changing* articles in the field of emergency medicine. We constructed this using a structured algorithm which drew on other rankings in the literature and on the rankings of each research study by the faculty of the Harvard Affiliated Emergency Medicine Residency.

There are many challenges inherent to creating any top 100 list. These studies have marked historical importance, and most have served as the foundation for further research. While we acknowledge that in many cases more recent studies have been published on the topic or review articles may be available, our goal is to make the original research that served as the bedrock for modern emergency medicine more accessible to the reader. Some of the studies included are negative studies. Understanding what was at the time a good idea but did not pan out as a therapy is just as important to our field as understanding what did work. Understanding why one intervention was better than another, or why one diagnostic test was chosen over another is critical to our growth as medical professionals and to developing the standard of care in our profession.

We recognize that many clinicians or researchers may disagree with the inclusion or exclusion of specific studies in our top 100 list. We understand and agree. We sought to identify studies that cover the broad scope of emergency care and the numerous patient populations cared for in the emergency department. If this book stimulates further discussion and critical debate regarding the published research, then we have achieved our purpose.

We hope you enjoy this book and that it helps with understanding why we do the things we do—the history and the science behind emergency medicine. Although the evidence will keep changing, and future editions will update this list, for now we offer this list and commentary as a starting point for those who want to understand the foundation of high-quality emergency care.

Emily L. Aaronson, MD
Erik L. Antonsen, MD, PhD
Arjun K. Venkatesh, MD, MBA, MHS

ACKNOWLEDGMENTS

The editors of this book are in debt to many people who helped make this happen. We would like to thank the Harvard Affiliated Emergency Medicine Residency Faculty who helped us distill our initial piles of papers into the list that appears in this book, especially Drs. Christopher Kabrhel, Toby Nagurney, Ali Raja, Lauren Allister, and Daniel Pallin. We would also like to thank Drs. Liu, Takayesu, Thomas, Soremekun, Duval, Levine, Tiamfook-Morgan for their dedication to creating the first HAEMR literature collection, which was one of several sources we drew upon to identify truly practice-changing studies in our field.

CONTENTS

SECTION 1: ABDOMINAL
Authors: Kathryn Hawk, Paulina B. Sergot

1. CT in the Diagnosis of Acute Appendicitis 2
2. Proton Pump Inhibitors in Bleeding Peptic Ulcer Disease..........................4
3. Somatostatin in Variceal Bleeding 6
4. Diagnostic Nasogastric Tubes in Hematemesis...8
5. Spontaneous Ureteral Stone Passage 10
6. Oral Ondansetron in Gastroenteritis 12
7. Oral vs. IV Rehydration 14

SECTION 2: AIRWAY
Authors: Andrew J. Eyre, Brock Daniels, Anita Rohra

8. Noninvasive Ventilation in Pulmonary Edema 18
9. End-tidal CO_2 in Sedation..20
10. RSI in ED Training 22
11. Hemoglobin Desaturation after Succinylcholine.......................................24
12. Laryngeal View Improvement in Laryngoscopy 26

SECTION 3: ALLERGY
Authors: Christina Wilson, Brock Daniels

13. Cephalosporins in Penicillin-allergic Patients 30
14. Histamine Antagonists in Acute Allergic Reaction 32

SECTION 4: CARDIOLOGY
Authors: Kenneth Bernard, Stephanie E. Burgos, Peter B. Pruitt Harman S. Gill, Joshua M. Keegan

15. TIMI Risk Score for ACS 36
16. Acute MI Without Chest Pain 38
17. Missed ACS in the ED 40
18. Troponins in Chest Pain 42
19. Beta-Blockers in Acute MI: The COMMIT Trial 44
20. Aspirin in Acute MI: The ISIS-2 Trial 46
21. Heparinizing Unstable Angina 48
22. Low-Molecular-Weight Heparin in Unstable Angina 50
23. tPA in Acute MI: The Gusto Trial 52
24. PCI vs. Lytics in Acute MI: The Gusto IIB Trial 54
25. PCI Timing in ACS 56
26. Delaying Defibrillation for CPR in Cardiac Arrest 58
27. Therapeutic Hypothermia in Cardiac Arrest 60
28. CPR Quality in Out-of-Hospital Cardiac Arrest 62
29. Chest Compression Only CPR 64
30. Amiodarone in Ventricular Fibrillation 66
31. Epinephrine in Cardiac Arrest 68
32. tPA in PEA Cardiac Arrest 70
33. Vasopressin vs. Epinephrine for Cardiac Arrest 72
34. Pill-in-the-Pocket Approach for Atrial Fibrillation 74
35. Rhythm Control in Atrial Fibrillation: The Affirm Trial 76
36. Risk of Stroke in Atrial Fibrillation Cardioversion 78

SECTION 5: ENDOCRINE
Author: Daphne Morrison Ponce

37. ABG vs. VBG in Diabetic Ketoacidosis 82
38. Bicarbonate Therapy in DKA 84

SECTION 6: INFECTIOUS DISEASE
Authors: Kito Lord, Ashley Kochanek, Jennifer Carnell

39. Early Goal-directed Therapy in Sepsis 88
40. The PORT Score 92
41. Steroids in Adult Meningitis 96
42. Steroids in Pediatric Meningitis 98
43. Doxycycline in Lyme Disease 100
44. An Intervention to Decrease Catheter-related Bloodstream Infection 102
45. Acute Otitis Media and Delayed Antibiotic Treatment 104
46. Centor Criteria for Strep Throat 106
47. The Febrile Infant 108
48. Risk of Serious Bacterial Infection in Febrile Infants with RSV 112

SECTION 7: NEUROLOGY
Authors: David Yamane, Michael E. Billington

49. CT Before Lumbar Puncture in Meningitis 116
50. Steroids and Antivirals in Bell's Palsy 118
51. Prochlorperazine in Migraine 120
52. Metoclopramide in Migraine 122
53. tPA for Acute Ischemic Stroke: The NINDS Trial 124
54. Intra-arterial tPA in Acute Ischemic Stroke: The Proact II Study 126
55. Timing of tPA in Acute Ischemic Stroke 128
56. Expanded Window for tPA in Stroke: The ECASS III Study 130
57. Determining Stroke Risk After TIA: The ABCD Score 132
58. Urgent Follow up for TIA: The EXPRESS Study 136
59. The Epley Maneuver for Vertigo 138
60. Risk of Seizure Recurrence in Pediatrics 140

SECTION 8: OPERATIONS
Authors: Christina Wilson, Ije Akunyili

61. Chest Pain Protocols in the ED 144
62. Stress Testing in the ED 146
63. Social Interventions for Alcohol Abuse 148

SECTION 9: ORTHOPEDICS
Author: Andrew J. Eyre

64. The Ottawa Knee Rules 152
65. The Ottawa Ankle Rules 154

SECTION 10: PAIN
Author: Michael E. Billington

66. Morphine and the Clinical Abdominal Exam 158
67. Ketorolac vs. Ibuprofen in Musculoskeletal Pain 160
68. Pain Management in the ED: The PEMI Study 162

SECTION 11: VENOUS THROMBOEMBOLISM
Author: Fan Yang

69. Clinical Diagnosis of PE 166
70. Prospective Evaluation of the PERC 168
71. D-Dimer in DVT and PE 172
72. V/Q Scan in Acute PE: The Pioped Trial 174
73. CT Imaging for Acute PE: The Pioped II Trial 176

SECTION 12: PSYCHIATRY
Author: Daphne Morrison Ponce

74. Pharmaceutical Restraints for Psychotic Agitation 180

SECTION 13: PULMONARY
Authors: Radhika Sundararajan, Joshua M. Keegan

75. Low Tidal Volume Ventilation in ARDS 184
76. Magnesium in Asthma 186
77. Dual Bronchodilators in Asthma 188
78. Dexamethasone for Croup 190
79. Oral vs. IV Steroids in COPD 192
80. Antibiotics in COPD Exacerbations 194
81. Pulse-Oximetry Replaces Arterial Blood Gases 196

SECTION 14: TOXICOLOGY
Authors: Sabrina J. Poon, Fan Yang, Spencer Greene, Silpa Gadiraju

82. Fomepizole in Ethylene Glycol Poisoning 200
83. Hyperbaric Oxygen in Carbon Monoxide Poisoning 202
84. The Rumack–Matthew Nomogram: Acetaminophen Poisoning and Toxicity...204
85. NAC in Acetaminophen Overdose 206
86. Cyanide Poisoning and Hydroxocobalamin..208
87. Digitalis Toxicity and Digoxin Immune Fab..210
88. Crofab in Snakebites 212

SECTION 15: TRAUMA
Authors: Andrew J. Eyre, Eva Tovar Hirashima, David Beversluis

89. Laparotomy in Abdominal Gunshot Wounds...216
90. Permissive Hypotension in Trauma 218
91. Level One Trauma Centers 220
92. CT vs. X-Ray in Traumatic Cervical Spine Injury 222
93. The NEXUS Criteria and the Canadian C-Spine Rules 224
94. New Orleans Criteria and the Canadian Head CT Rules 228
95. ED Thoracotomies 232
96. Pediatric Head Trauma 234

SECTION 16: ULTRASOUND
Authors: Christina Wilson, Daphne Morrison Ponce

97. Point of Care Echo in Penetrating Cardiac Injury..................................238
98. The Importance of Ultrasound in Central Venous Line Placement.........240
99. Ultrasound in Trauma...242
100. Ultrasound for Resuscitation Termination 244

INDEX **247**

SECTION 1: ABDOMINAL

Kathryn Hawk ■ Paulina B. Sergot

1. CT in the Diagnosis of Acute Appendicitis
2. Proton Pump Inhibitors in Bleeding Peptic Ulcer Disease
3. Somatostatin in Variceal Bleeding
4. Diagnostic Nasogastric Tubes in Hematemesis
5. Spontaneous Ureteral Stone Passage
6. Oral Ondansetron in Gastroenteritis
7. Oral vs. IV Rehydration

CT IN THE DIAGNOSIS OF ACUTE APPENDICITIS

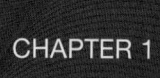

Effect of Computed Tomography of the Appendix on Treatment of Patients and Use of Hospital Resources
Rao PM, Rhea JT, Novelline RA, et al. *NEJM.* 1998;338(3):141–146

BACKGROUND
In 1994 ACEP released clinical guidelines for the workup of suspected appendicitis, which included complete blood count (CBC), urinalysis, consult, and admission.[1] The diagnosis of appendicitis was a clinical diagnosis confirmed only by pathology or the test of time. Prior to the widespread use of CT scan, patients with suspected appendicitis were taken directly to the operating room or hospitalized for serial abdominal examinations, often resulting in potentially avoidable hospital admissions. Prior to imaging it was estimated that a significant number of appendicitis cases were missed and 15% of patients who underwent surgery had a normal appendix.[2]

OBJECTIVES
To determine if the routine use of appendiceal CT scan in patients with suspected appendicitis changes patient care and its impact on hospital resources.

METHODS
Prospective, observational, single-center study conducted in the United States in 1996.

Participants
One hundred consecutive patients in whom a surgeon recommended hospital admission for observation or emergent appendectomy based on history, physical examination, and laboratory data. Patients who were pregnant were excluded.

Intervention Evaluated
Routine appendiceal CT in the ED for patients with planned hospitalization for suspected appendicitis or urgent appendectomy.

Outcomes
Changes in patient care and the costs of appendectomy, negative appendectomy, hospital days, and CT scan were estimated based on recent hospital data.

KEY RESULTS
- CT scan results changed the medical management of 59 patients, preventing 13 unnecessary appendectomies and avoiding 50 patient-days of unnecessary hospital admission.
- Forty-seven patients were determined not to have a clinical diagnosis of appendicitis based on negative appendectomy (3), other surgery (3), or clinical follow-up (41).

- The interpretation of appendiceal CT scans was 98% sensitive and 98% specific (based on pathology confirmation).
- The estimated hospital cost was lowest for patients who underwent appendiceal CT scan ($228 vs. $405 for 1 day of observation for low-acuity patient vs. $3,637 for unnecessary appendectomy).
- The overall cost savings was $447 per patient.

STUDY FINDINGS

The routine use of appendiceal CT in the ED for patients in whom appendicitis is clinically suspected is cost-effective and improves patient care by avoiding unnecessary hospitalization and surgical intervention.

COMMENTARY

Prior to this study CT scans were increasingly available in the ED and considered an extravagant imaging modality with unclear diagnostic utility. Estimating and evaluating the costs of the treatment plan before and after CT scan allowed a direct comparison of associated costs and made a compelling case for the routine use of CT scans in patients with suspected appendicitis. These findings should be interpreted with some caution as this study used appendiceal CT scan that used rectal contrast and was completed within 1 hour of ordering—none of which reflect the current use of multidetector CT in the ED. This article supports the routine use of appendiceal CT scan in patients with suspected appendicitis as an accurate and cost-effective clinical tool, and was cited in the 2000 ACEP clinical guidelines on the evaluation and management of ED patients with nontraumatic abdominal pain.[3] This shift in clinical practice set the stage for the more widespread use of CT scan for the evaluation of acute abdominal pain across a wider range of diagnoses with similar impacts on hospitalization.

Question
Does CT imaging improve outcomes for patients with suspected appendicitis?

Answer
Yes, the use of CT imaging can reduce hospitalizations, negative appendectomies, and cost.

References
1. Clinical policy for the initial approach to patients presenting with a chief complaint of nontraumatic acute abdominal pain. *Ann Emerg Med.* 1994;23(4):906–922.
2. Drake F, et al. Progress in the Diagnosis of Appendicitis: A Report from Washington State's Surgical Care and Outcomes Assessment Program (SCOAP). *Ann Surg.* 2012;256(4):586–594.
3. Clinical policy: Critical issues for the initial evaluation and management of patients presenting with a chief complaint of nontraumatic acute abdominal pain. *Ann Emerg Med.* 2000;36(4):406–415.

CHAPTER 2: PROTON PUMP INHIBITORS IN BLEEDING PEPTIC ULCER DISEASE

A Comparison of Omeprazole and Placebo for Bleeding Peptic Ulcer
Khuroo MS, Yattoo GN, Javid G, et al. *NEJM*. 1997;336(15):1054–1058

BACKGROUND
At the time of this article, endoscopic techniques were widely used to treat patients bleeding from a peptic ulcer. However, no specific medical therapy had been shown to be effective as an alternative for controlling ulcer-related hemorrhage and decreasing its recurrence. As platelet function is severely impaired at high pH in vitro, a potential strategy was to reduce gastric acidity to a nearly neutral pH, which could stabilize the clot over the ulcer and stop bleeding or prevent recurrence.

OBJECTIVES
To investigate whether administering a proton pump inhibitor (PPI) will stop bleeding or prevent recurrent bleeding in peptic ulcer disease (PUD).

METHODS
Double-blinded, randomized control trial at a single center between 1992 and 1994.

Patients
Eight hundred and sixty patients presenting with upper gastrointestinal bleeding underwent emergency endoscopy within 12 hours of presentation, and 680 were found to have PUD. Of these, 220 patients had stigmata of active or recent hemorrhage and were randomized immediately after performance of endoscopy. Select exclusion criteria: Patients presenting with a contraindication to endoscopy or those requiring immediate surgery.

Interventions
Omeprazole 40 mg or placebo administered orally every 12 hours for 5 days. No intravenous (IV) formulation was available.

Outcomes
The primary outcomes were rate of further or recurrent bleeding, need for surgical intervention, and mortality related to bleeding or treatment received within 30 days of admission. Secondary outcomes included need for blood transfusion and length of stay in the hospital.

KEY RESULTS
- Rate of continued or further bleeding was significantly lower in the omeprazole group compared to placebo (10.9% vs. 36.4%), as was the need for surgical intervention (7.3% vs. 23.6%).

- There was little difference in the mortality between groups (1.8% vs. 5.5%).
- Significantly fewer patients in the treatment group received blood transfusions (29.1% vs. 70.9%), and these patients had significantly shorter hospital lengths of stay (5.5 ± 2.1 vs. 6.9 ± 2.1 days).

STUDY CONCLUSIONS

Omeprazole therapy was associated with significant reductions in the rates of further bleeding and surgical intervention, the number of days in the hospital, and the need for blood transfusion in bleeding PUD.

COMMENTARY

Prior to this study, H_2-receptor blockers had been investigated but had not demonstrated a treatment benefit in upper gastrointestinal bleeding. In addition, one large trial of omeprazole did not show any benefit, but it included all patients with upper gastrointestinal bleeding, regardless of cause or risk factors. This study narrowed the population to those with bleeding peptic ulcers and was pivotal in establishing a role for proton pump inhibition in decreasing recurrent bleeding, possibly due to the neutralizing effect on gastric pH. It is important to note that this study did not evaluate the potential benefit of combining omeprazole with endoscopic therapy. Based on these findings and subsequent trials, published guidelines recommend PPI therapy in patients with upper gastrointestinal bleeding. Although it has become routine to administer an IV bolus of 80 mg of a proton pump inhibitor followed by a continuous infusion of 8 mg per hour, the route of administration, dosage, timing with endoscopy, and patient population most likely to benefit are still under investigation.

Question

Is the administration of omeprazole beneficial to patients presenting with bleeding peptic ulcer disease?

Answer

Yes, oral omeprazole can decrease the rate of further bleeding, surgical interventions, blood transfusions, and hospital length of stay.

CHAPTER 3

SOMATOSTATIN IN VARICEAL BLEEDING

Early Administration of Vapreotide for Variceal Bleeding in Patients with Cirrhosis
Calès P, Masliah C, Bernard B, et al. *NEJM*. 2001;344(1):23–28

BACKGROUND
Mortality from a single episode of esophageal variceal bleeding ranges from 10% to 70% depending on the degree of underlying liver dysfunction.[1] It is critical to stop acute bleeding and to prevent rebleeding after sclerotherapy, but research results regarding the benefit of adding a somatostatin analog were mixed. One 1995 study showed that the combination of the somatostatin analog octreotide and sclerotherapy was more effective than sclerotherapy alone in the control of acute variceal bleeding, though overall mortality was not affected.[2] Prior to this study, patients were frequently treated with both somatostatin analogs and endoscopic therapy, although the overall benefit of somatostatin analogs and the need of early administration were unclear.

OBJECTIVES
To determine if the administration of vapreotide prior to endoscopy affected the control of variceal bleeding, the rate of early recurrence, or 42-day mortality.

METHODS
Double-blinded prospective randomized control trial at 22 medical centers between 1997 and 1998.

Patients
Two hundred and twenty-seven patients, between 18 and 75 years old, with documented cirrhosis and acute onset variceal bleeding. Inclusion criteria: Child–Pugh score of less than 13, and an initial onset of bleeding <24 hours prior to enrollment. Select exclusion criteria: A patent shunt, known hepatocellular carcinoma or complete portal vein thrombosis, coma, pregnant or breast-feeding, or variceal bleed within preceding 6 weeks.

Interventions
Patients were enrolled within 6 hours of hospital admission and were randomized to receive either vapreotide or placebo prior to endoscopic intervention.

Outcomes
The primary outcome of the study was the combined outcome of control of bleeding (absence of bleeding at 6 and 48 hours after endoscopy) and survival at 5 days. Secondary outcomes included control of bleeding during initial endoscopic procedure (an average of 2.6 hours ± 3.3 hours after initiation of infusion), 5- and 42-day mortality and number of units of packed red blood cells (pRBCs) to maintain hematocrit (HCT) >27.

KEY RESULTS
- Control of bleeding and survival at day 5 was higher in the vapreotide group compared to the control (66% vs. 50%).
- Control of bleeding achieved on initial endoscopy was higher in the vapreotide group compared to the control (69% vs. 54%); $p = 0.03$.
- The vapreotide group required significantly fewer transfusions (2 ± 2.2 vs. 2.8 ± 2.8 units) to maintain a HCT >27 ($p = 0.04$).
- Early (day 3 to 5) and late (day 6 to 42) recurrent bleeding was rare and did not differ between groups.
- Five- and 42-day mortality did not differ between groups according to Kaplan-Meier estimates.

STUDY CONCLUSIONS
In cirrhotic patients with acute onset variceal bleeding, the administration of vapreotide followed by endoscopic intervention improves the combined outcome of 5-day survival with control of bleeding. Vapreotide administration also results in fewer blood transfusions, though overall (noncombined outcome) mortality at 5 and 42 days was not affected.

COMMENTARY
In part because of the significant mortality associated with variceal bleeding, somatostatin analogs were frequently administered despite the unclear effect of these agents on clinical outcomes. This study added to earlier observations that the use of vasoactive somatostatin analog prior to early endoscopic intervention improves the likelihood of early control of acute variceal bleeding. Of note, both the control and treatment groups received antibiotic prophylaxis, which in combination with somatostatin analogs and endoscopic intervention continues to be the standard of care. Readers should remember that the outcome measures only included short-term 5-day mortality and that the study does not report pre- or procedural use of proton pump inhibitors, which may have also confounded these results. Results of this and other work prompted the first of several Baveno consensus conferences, which provided diagnostic and management recommendations for variceal bleeding, consistent definitions for use in research studies, and directions for future clinical trials.[3]

Question
Should somatostatin analogs be given to patients with suspected variceal bleeding?

Answer
Yes, somatostatin analogs prior to endoscopy can decrease the need for blood transfusions.

References
1. *World Gastroenterology Organization Practice Guideline: Esophageal Varices.* June 2008.
2. Besson I, Ingrand P, Person B, et al. Sclerotherapy with or without octreotide for acute variceal bleeding. *N Engl J Med.* 1995;333:555–560.
3. Bari K, Garcia-Tsao G. Treatment of portal hypertension. *World J Gastroenterol.* 2012;18(11):1166–1175.

CHAPTER 4
DIAGNOSTIC NASOGASTRIC TUBES IN HEMATEMESIS

Usefulness and Validity of Diagnostic Nasogastric Aspiration in Patients Without Hematemesis
Witting MD, Magder L, Heins AE, et al. *Ann Emerg Med.* 2004;43:525–532

BACKGROUND
GI bleeding is a common ED presentation with significant associated morbidity and mortality. It is often difficult to distinguish upper and lower GI sources of bleeding, though this can have significant treatment implications. Nasogastric (NG) aspiration has long been thought of as one way to emergently differentiate upper and lower sources of GI bleeding. At the time of this study, it was not known whether knowledge gained from NG aspiration actually influences emergent management and outweighs patient discomfort and complications, such as tube misplacement and aspiration.

OBJECTIVES
To estimate the test characteristics (sensitivity, specificity, positive predictive value [PPV], negative predictive value [NPV], likelihood ratio [LR]) of NG aspiration to diagnose upper GI bleed in ED patients without hematemesis.

METHODS
Retrospective cohort study at two urban hospitals between 1997 and 2002.

Patients
Two hundred and twenty adult patients with dark, black or bloody stools and confirmatory diagnostic testing within 3 days of ED presentation. Select exclusion criteria: Patients with hematemesis, an obvious source of anorectal bleeding, ostomy, or hospital admission for GI bleeding in the previous month.

Interventions
NG lavage was performed on all patients. The results of NG aspiration were abstracted from the chart by two abstractors to ensure reliability. All results were classified by a six-category classification system ranging from clearly negative to clearly positive. Test characteristics, including sensitivity and specificity were calculated based on the discharge ICD-9 code in conjunction with gastroenterologist documentation and confirmatory testing.

Outcomes
The primary outcome was the specificity, sensitivity, PPV, NPV, and LR of NG aspiration detection of upper GI bleeding in patients with evidence of GI bleed without hematemesis, using confirmatory testing within 3 days as a reference standard.

KEY RESULTS
- NG aspiration was 42% sensitive and 91% specific for detecting upper GI bleeding.
- The negative predictive value was 64% and the positive predictive value was 92%.
- The likelihood ratio of a positive nasogastric aspiration was 11 and the likelihood ratio of a negative nasogastric aspiration was 0.6.
- Patients offered NG aspiration had a lower frequency of bright red blood per rectum, a lower median hematocrit, and were more likely to receive a final diagnosis of upper GI hemorrhage than those not offered lavage.
- Ninety-eight percent (48/49) of patients with a positive NG lavage underwent confirmatory esophagogastroduodenoscopy (EGD) whereas 61% (97/158) of patients with a negative NG lavage had an EGD.

STUDY CONCLUSIONS
A positive NG aspiration, as seen in 23% of patients in this study, was highly suggestive of an upper GI source (LR 11), but a negative aspiration provides little information.

COMMENTARY
The ability to differentiate a Upper gastrointestinal bleed (UGIB) from a lower gastrointestinal bleed (LGIB) is highly desirable given the possibility of deferring an EGD; however the primary test available, NG lavage, had exceedingly variable effectiveness and reliability. The results of this study demonstrate the utility of a positive NG aspiration in patients with GI bleeding, though that result was evident in less than 25% of patients who underwent the procedure. An important point that is not addressed by this study is whether or not the results of the aspiration significantly change patient management, as 61% of patients with a negative lavage still had a confirmatory EGD. This study does show that NG aspiration can be a useful test, although the overall utility of the NG lavage with respect to subsequent management appears minimal based on more recent clinical studies.

Question
Is nasogastric aspiration a useful test in detecting upper gastrointestinal (GI) bleeding in patients without hematemesis?

Answer
Perhaps, a negative lavage is not sufficiently sensitive to exclude an upper GI bleed, and a positive lavage, while highly specific for an upper GI bleed, is unlikely to alter clinical management as nearly all of these patients will receive subsequent endoscopy.

CHAPTER 5
SPONTANEOUS URETERAL STONE PASSAGE

Relationship of Spontaneous Passage of Ureteral Calculi to Stone Size and Location as Revealed by Unenhanced Helical CT
Coll DM, Varanelli MJ, Smith RC. *AJR Am J Roentgenol.* 2002;178:101–103

BACKGROUND
When clinicians diagnose ureterolithiasis in the ED, patients frequently ask "Will this go away on its own?" Prior to this study, the bulk of the data surrounding spontaneous passage of ureteral stones was based on radiography, which was less sensitive for detecting stones and did not account for radiolucent stones, such as those made of uric acid or xanthine. As unenhanced CT imaging began to play a larger role in the diagnosis of ureterolithiasis it was not known if current urologic guidelines on the spontaneous passage of stones would be affected by the use of a more sensitive diagnostic test.

OBJECTIVES
To determine the relationship between size and location of ureterolithiasis as seen on unenhanced CT scan in relation to likelihood of spontaneous passage.

METHODS
Retrospective observational study between 1994 and 1996.

Patients
Participants included 172 adults with solitary ureteral stone seen on unenhanced CT independently confirmed by other imaging studies, interventional procedures, or documented clinical follow-up. Neither the characteristics of patients who received intervention nor the setting in which the CT scan was ordered was reported. Select exclusion criteria were not reported.

Intervention
To examine the relationship between size and location of ureteral stone as seen on unenhanced CT scan and spontaneous passage. Fifty-seven of the 172 patients received interventional therapy based on patient specific factors including pain tolerance and concern for infection.

Outcomes
The primary outcome was the relationship of ureteral stone size and location as seen on unenhanced CT to the probability of spontaneous passage.

KEY RESULTS
- The overall frequency of spontaneous passage was 78% for 1 to 4 mm stones, 60% for 5 to 7 mm stones, and 39% for stones >8 mm.
- The overall frequency of stone passage was 48% for proximal stones, 60% for midureteral stones, 75% for distal stones, and 79% for stones located at the ureterovesical junction.
- When evaluating likelihood of spontaneous passage of the size of stones at specific anatomical location, the only statistically significant relationship found was for stones at the ureterovesical junction.

STUDY CONCLUSIONS
The likelihood of spontaneous passage of ureteral stones varies with size and location as seen on CT scan, and is similar to previous results based on radiography.

COMMENTARY
In the era of increased CT scan utilization for the diagnosis of ureterolithiasis, this study aimed to determine the relationship of ureteral stones' size and location and the likelihood of spontaneous passage. They reported an almost linear correlation between size and likelihood of spontaneous passage of stone and found an inverse relationship between proximal location and likelihood of spontaneous passage. These findings were not only consistent with previous data based on radiography, but also more generalizable given the precision with which stone location and size can be determined with CT. Of note, this study did not exclusively enroll ED patients, though the results are likely generalizable to the ED patient population. This study enabled clinicians to better inform patients and pursue a conservative outpatient management plan rather than favoring consultation for intervention in smaller more distal stones.

Question
Does the size and location of a kidney stone identified on CT imaging predict clinically meaningful outcomes?

Answer
Yes, smaller and more distally located stones have a higher likelihood of spontaneous passage without intervention.

CHAPTER 6
ORAL ONDANSETRON IN GASTROENTERITIS

Oral Ondansetron for Gastroenteritis in a Pediatric Emergency Department
Freedman SB, Adler M, Seshadri R, et al. *N Engl J Med.* 2006;354(16):1698–1705

BACKGROUND
Gastroenteritis is a common presentation of pediatric patients in the ED and accounts for more than 1.5 million outpatient visits and 200,000 hospitalizations annually.[1] Oral rehydration for patients with mild-to-moderate dehydration is recommended as the preferred therapy by the Center for Disease Control (CDC) and the American Academy of Pediatrics (AAP), but is not always practiced as clinicians are often reticent to use oral rehydration in patients with recent history of vomiting.[2] At the time of this study, ondansetron was a potent new antiemetic that had not been studied as an adjunct to oral rehydration.

OBJECTIVES
To determine if oral ondansetron decreased vomiting or improved clinical outcomes in patients receiving oral rehydration therapy for mild-to-moderate dehydration as a result of gastroenteritis.

METHODS
Prospective, double-blind, randomized controlled trial conducted in an academic pediatric ED between 2004 and 2005.

Patients
Two hundred and fifteen children between the ages of 6 months and 10 years who presented to the ED with at least one episode of nonbloody, nonbilious emesis within the preceding 4 hours, at least one episode of diarrhea during their illness, and a dehydration score consistent with mild-to-moderate dehydration. Select exclusion criteria: Evidence of severe dehydration and weight <8 kg.

Interventions
Patients were randomized to receive ondansetron or placebo. Both groups received an initial weight-based dose (ondansetron or placebo) followed by a second dose if the patient vomited within 15 minutes of the first dose. A 1-hour period of intense oral rehydration was initiated 15 minutes after the intervention, and oral rehydration therapy was continued until appropriate disposition was determined. Patients were followed up by telephone 3 and 7 days postintervention.

Outcomes
The primary outcome was vomiting while receiving oral rehydration therapy. Secondary outcomes included the number of episodes of vomiting during oral rehydration therapy, rates of IV hydration as a rescue therapy, and hospitalization.

KEY RESULTS
- Vomiting during oral rehydration occurred significantly less in the ondansetron group when compared to placebo (14% vs. 35%; RR = 0.40).
- Children who received ondansetron had less vomiting (0.18 vs. 0.65 episodes), greater oral intake (239 mL vs. 196 mL), and were less likely to receive IV hydration (14% vs. 31%, RR 0.46).
- There was no significant difference in the rates of hospitalizations or return visits.
- The mean length of stay was 12% shorter in the ondansetron group ($p = 0.02$).

STUDY CONCLUSIONS
A single dose of ondansetron in pediatric ED patients with mild-to-moderate dehydration from gastroenteritis decreases vomiting and facilitates oral hydration.

COMMENTARY

Despite AAP and CDC recommendations for oral rehydration therapy in mild-to-moderate dehydration, many pediatricians and emergency physicians favored IV rehydration in this population, with vomiting being an often-cited explanation.[1,2] The results of this study confirm that vomiting is not a contraindication to oral rehydration and that the administration of a single oral dose of ondansetron improves the success of oral rehydration therapy and other clinical outcomes. A 2011 Cochrane review of seven trials confirmed these findings and showed that oral ondansetron increased the proportion of patients who had ceased vomiting and reduced the number needing IV rehydration and immediate hospital admission.[3] These findings have had wider adoption in resource-limited global settings, as well as in pediatric settings seeking to minimize invasive and painful IV placement, but are yet to be adopted broadly in adult EDs.

Question
Does ondansetron improve outcomes in patients with mild-to-moderate dehydration due to gastroenteritis?

Answer
Yes, a single dose of ondansetron decreases vomiting during oral rehydration and the need for IV hydration although it may not affect rates of hospitalization.

References
1. Practice parameter: The management of acute gastroenteritis in young children. *Pediatrics.* 1996;97(3):424–435.
2. Ozuah PO, Avner JR, Stein RE. Oral rehydration, emergency physicians, and practice parameters: A national survey. *Pediatrics.* 2002;109:259–261.
3. Fedorowicz Z, Jagannath VA, Carter B. Antiemetics for reducing vomiting related to acute gastroenteritis in children and adolescents. *Cochrane Database Syst Rev.* 2011;(9):CD005506.

CHAPTER 7   ORAL VS. IV REHYDRATION

Oral vs. Intravenous Rehydration of Moderately Dehydrated Children: A Randomized, Controlled trial.

Spandorfer PR, Alessandrini EA, Joffe MD, et al. Pediatrics. 2005;115(2):295–301

BACKGROUND
Despite guidelines recommending that oral rehydration therapy (ORT) is the recommended first-line treatment for mild and moderate dehydration due to gastroenteritis, a 2002 survey found that 75% of clinicians with endorsed knowledge of these guidelines almost exclusively used intravenous (IV) hydration.[1] A multitude of factors have been cited as potential sources of this discrepancy including beliefs about parents' expectations, the presence of vomiting, and the time and resources involved in administering oral rehydration. This study aimed to elucidate the failure rates of ORT and to evaluate the overall impact of ORT on hospital resources and patient experience.

OBJECTIVES
To determine whether the failure rate of ORT in moderately dehydrated patients would be less than 5% of the failure rate observed in patients who received IV hydration.

METHODS
Randomized, controlled, single-blind, noninferiority study conducted at an urban tertiary children's hospital ED from 2001 to 2003.

Patients
Seventy-three patients aged 8 weeks to 3 years old with a diagnosis of probable viral gastroenteritis and moderate dehydration. Select exclusion criteria: Hypotension, duration of illness >5 days, other recent ED treatment, and underlying medical problems that impact fluid status.

Interventions
Pedialyte ORT in fixed aliquots over 4 hours compared with IV normal saline and ORT combined. Evaluating physicians were blinded. The 36 patients in the ORT group received Pedialyte in fixed aliquots over 4 hours and sham IV placement.

Outcomes
The primary outcome was success of ED treatment at 4 hours, which was defined as resolution of moderate dehydration (dehydration score ≤2), weight gain, production of urine during the trial, and absence of severe emesis (≥5 mL/kg) during the last hour. Predefined secondary outcomes were time to initiation of therapy, improvement of dehydration score at 2 hours, hospitalization rate, 72 hour returns, and parental preference for the same therapy at 4 hours.

KEY RESULTS
- Successful rehydration at 4 hours was equal in both groups (55.6% of the oral rehydration group and 56.8% in the IV hydration group).
- The mean time to treatment onset was 21.2 minutes shorter in the ORT group (19.9 vs. 41.2 minutes in IV hydration group).
- More patients in the IV hydration group were hospitalized (48.7% vs. 30.6% in the ORT group).
- No difference was seen in dehydration score at 2 hours, parental preference for the same therapy next time, or 72-hour returns.

STUDY CONCLUSIONS
ORT is not inferior to IV hydration for the treatment of moderate dehydration in those with a presumed diagnosis of gastroenteritis. Time to initiation of treatment was significantly faster in the oral rehydration group.

COMMENTARY
Despite recommendations by the Center for Disease Control, the American Academy of Pediatrics, and the World Health Organization, the practice of ORT for the treatment of moderate dehydration remains varied. The goal of this study was to show that ORT did not result in more treatment failures than IV hydration, and to explore specific concerns that had been cited as reasons for choosing IV over oral hydration. Although follow-up studies are needed to evaluate cost and generalizability, this study used rigorous methodology to minimize bias and made a compelling argument for the first-line use of oral rehydration in patients with moderate dehydration due to gastroenteritis. A 2010 publication by the ACEP Pediatric Emergency Medicine Committee concluded that oral rehydration is highly effective, safe, and inexpensive and the available evidence supports ORT in the majority of children with gastroenteritis and mild-to-moderate dehydration.[2]

Question
Is oral rehydration as effective as IV hydration in moderately dehydrated patients due to gastroenteritis?

Answer
Yes, both oral and IV rehydration showed the same improvement in dehydration scores during a 4-hour ED visit.

References
1. Ozuah PO, Avner JR, Stein RE. Oral Rehydration, Emergency Physicians, and practice parameters: A national survey. *Pediatrics.* 2002;109:259–261.
2. Colletti JE, Brown KM, Sharieff GQ, Barata IA, Ishimine P; ACEP Pediatric Emergency Medicine Committee. The management of children with gastroenteritis and dehydration in the emergency department. *J Emerg Med.* 2010;38(5):686–698.

SECTION 2: AIRWAY

Andrew J. Eyre ■ Brock Daniels ■ Anita Rohra

8. Noninvasive Ventilation in Pulmonary Edema
9. End-tidal CO_2 in Sedation
10. RSI in ED Training
11. Hemoglobin Desaturation after Succinylcholine
12. Laryngeal View Improvement in Laryngoscopy

CHAPTER 8
NONINVASIVE VENTILATION IN PULMONARY EDEMA

Efficacy and Safety of Non-invasive Ventilation in the Treatment of Acute Cardiogenic Pulmonary Edema – A Systemic Review and Meta-analysis
Winck JC, Azevedo LF, Costa-Pereira A, et al. *Crit Care.* 2006;10(2):R69

BACKGROUND
Heart failure and acute pulmonary edema are frequent reasons for ED admission, and heart failure is the most common cause of hospital admission in patients over 65. These diseases are associated with high mortality and appropriate treatment can be resource intensive and expensive. Both continuous positive airway pressure ventilation (CPAP) and noninvasive positive pressure ventilation (NPPV or BiPAP) had become critical tools in the treatment of these patients; however, at the time of this meta-analysis several studies had left important unanswered questions: One showed that CPAP decreased the need for endotracheal intubation but had no effect on mortality while another suggested that NPPV may be associated with increased incidence of acute myocardial infarction (AMI).

OBJECTIVES
To evaluate the efficacy of CPAP and NPPV in patients with acute pulmonary edema based on three outcomes: The need for intubation, overall mortality, and incidence of AMI.

METHODS
A systematic literature review of randomized control trials published through May of 2005. Of the 790 articles originally considered, 17 were used in the final analysis.

Participants
Most studies were small, with a median of 40 patients per study in the 17 original articles (range 22 to 130). A total of 938 patients were represented.

Interventions
The use of CPAP or NPPV compared to standard medical therapy in 10 of the studies; the other seven either compared CPAP to NPPV directly, or were three-armed comparing both to standard medical therapy.

Outcomes
Need for endotracheal intubation, all-cause in-hospital mortality, and risk of AMI.

KEY RESULTS
- CPAP had a 22% absolute risk reduction in the need for endotracheal intubation and a 13% absolute risk reduction in mortality.

- NPPV had an 18% absolute risk reduction in the need for endotracheal intubation and a nonsignificant 7% absolute risk reduction in mortality.
- There was no significant difference in the need for intubation or mortality between CPAP and NPPV.
- There was no significant increase in the risk for AMI with CPAP or NPPV when compared to standard medical therapy.

STUDY CONCLUSIONS

CPAP and NPPV both greatly decrease mortality and need for intubation in patients with acute pulmonary edema without a significant difference between them. There is no increased risk of AMI. CPAP is less expensive and easier to use than NPPV.

COMMENTARY

This comprehensive meta-analysis leveraged a number of small studies and uncovered the benefits of, and differences between, CPAP and NPPV. Ultimately, the study finds that there is no significant difference between CPAP and NPPV and that either intervention can effectively reduce the need for intubation and decrease mortality in patients with acute pulmonary edema. While many hospitals continue to employ NPPV as the modality of choice for patients presenting with acute pulmonary edema, CPAP is as safe and effective and its use should be encouraged in the prehospital setting and in EDs without advanced respiratory capabilities.

Question

Is there a difference between CPAP and BiPAP with regard to safety or efficacy?

Answer

No, both forms of noninvasive ventilation reduce mortality and the need for intubation in patients with pulmonary edema without increasing the risk of acute MI. CPAP is easier and less expensive to use.

CHAPTER 9 END-TIDAL CO_2 IN SEDATION

Does End-tidal Carbon Dioxide Monitoring Detect Respiratory Events Prior to Current Sedation Monitoring Practices?
Burton JH, Harrah JD, Germann CA, et al. *Acad Emerg Med.* 2006;13(5):500–504

BACKGROUND
End-tidal carbon dioxide ($ETCO_2$) monitoring is the standard of care in the operating room for monitoring of ventilation, and is the fastest known indicator for apnea, respiratory depression, and airway compromise. Pulse oximetry, the standard of care in the ED prior to this study, is known to have a 2- to 3-minute delay in detecting hypoxemia. Procedural sedation and analgesia (PSA) in the ED can lead to airway compromise and requires continuous monitoring of vital signs. Prior to this study, no specialty organization recommended the routine use of $ETCO_2$ in the ED.

OBJECTIVES
To determine if $ETCO_2$ monitoring during PSA in the ED accurately detected acute respiratory events before current methods.

METHODS
Prospective observational study, convenience sample, in 2004.

Participants
Fifty-nine patients undergoing 60 PSA encounters who presented when a study investigator was available were enrolled over a 6-month period.

Interventions
Standard monitoring (continuous SpO_2, heart rate, respiratory rate, rhythm, and interval blood pressure) and $ETCO_2$ monitoring was performed on all PSA patients. Physicians involved in care were blinded to interval $ETCO_2$ readings recorded by a study investigator. All patients were administered supplemental oxygen at 2 L/min in concordance with the institutional PSA policy.

Outcomes
The primary outcome was acute respiratory event, defined as oxygen saturation <92%, increase in oxygen provided due to observed apnea, hypoventilation, use of bag valve mask (BVM) or nasal/oral airway, physical or verbal stimulation, or use of a reversal agent. Change in $ETCO_2$ >10 mm Hg from baseline and $ETCO_2$ <30 mm Hg or >50 mm Hg were also considered acute respiratory events.

KEY RESULTS
- Abnormal $ETCO_2$ levels were documented in 60% of PSA encounters.
- In 44% of those with abnormal $ETCO_2$ levels, no acute respiratory event was observed requiring intervention.
- Eighty-five percent of patients with acute respiratory events had abnormal $ETCO_2$ values.
- Seventy percent of patients with acute respiratory events had abnormal $ETCO_2$ values prior to standard indicators.
- Despite original plans of enrolling 250 patients for the study, it was determined that the study should be terminated after 60 patients so that all patients having PSA could have nonblinded $ETCO_2$ monitoring.

STUDY CONCLUSIONS
$ETCO_2$ monitoring detected many clinically relevant acute respiratory events during PSA encounters. The majority of these events were detected by $ETCO_2$ prior to standard monitoring.

COMMENTARY
This study was performed to determine the utility of $ETCO_2$ monitoring during PSA encounters in the ED. It demonstrated that the majority of acute respiratory events can be detected by $ETCO_2$ monitoring prior to standard monitoring, and that the differences detected were so robust that early termination of the study was required to ensure broader application of this approach. Subsequent clinical guidelines support $ETCO_2$ monitoring during PSA in the ED.[1] This study did not show that the earlier detection of an acute respiratory event translated into an intervention that lessened the severity or prevented it altogether, but the potential for this exists with a relatively harmless and inexpensive intervention, highlighting the greater significance of this study. These findings have also helped broaden the use of $ETCO_2$ monitoring in predicting acute respiratory events in the prehospital settings and in patients with acute respiratory failure.

Question
Should end-tidal capnography be used during procedural sedation in the ED?

Answer
Yes, capnography can detect respiratory events during procedural sedation earlier than standard monitoring procedures.

Reference
1. Clinical Policy: Procedural Sedation and Analgesia in the Emergency Department, ACEP Clinical Policies Subcommittee on Procedural Sedation and Analgesia. *Ann Emerg Med.* 2014;63:247–258.

CHAPTER 10 RSI IN ED TRAINING

Rapid-sequence Intubation at an Emergency Medicine Residency: Success Rate and Adverse Events During a Two-year Period
Tayal VS, Riggs RW, Marx JA, et al. *Acad Emerg Med.* 1999;6(1):31–37

BACKGROUND
During the 1980s and early 1990s the use of neuromuscular blocking agents for rapid sequence intubation (RSI) was demonstrated to improve intubation success rates and outcomes for patients requiring airway management in the ED. While prior studies had shown that RSI was safe and effective in community EDs, little published data existed to support the safe use of RSI by EM trainees. Institutional and interdepartmental resistance to the use of paralytics by EM trainees persisted, in part due to this knowledge gap.

OBJECTIVES
To evaluate the rate of successful intubation, as well as major adverse events, related to RSI in an EM residency program.

METHODS
Observational study conducted at an urban, tertiary care ED and Level I trauma center with an EM training program between 1993 and 1994.

Participants
Four hundred and seventeen consecutive patients presenting to the ED requiring RSI (48% were medical, 44% trauma, and 8% toxicologic). Operators were 22 board-certified EM faculty and 30 EM residents (PGY 1 to 3). Residents were required to take an annual airway management course as part of their curriculum.

Intervention
Data was collected on the number of attempts at endotracheal intubation, training level of operator, type of definitive airway ultimately secured and by whom, RSI medications given and adverse events. Intubations were performed using induction and neuromuscular blocking agents chosen by the treating clinicians.

Outcomes
The primary outcome was intubation success rate. Secondary outcomes included the number of adverse events related to RSI. Major adverse events were defined as occurring within 10 minutes of RSI and included one or more of the following: Desaturation to oxygen saturation <90% (hypoxemia), decrease in systolic blood pressure <90 mm Hg for >10 minutes, any decrease in blood pressure requiring initiation of vasopressor support (hypotension), or any dysrhythmia.

KEY RESULTS
- Successful tracheal intubation was accomplished in one or two attempts in 96.5% of patients.
- Major immediate adverse events occurred in 1.4% (6) of cases including hypotension (2), hypoxemia (1), and dysrhythmia (3). No deaths were attributed to RSI performed by emergency physicians in the ED.
- Midazolam was the most common induction agent (50%), followed by thiopental (21%). Succinylcholine was used in 96% of cases.

STUDY CONCLUSIONS
RSI can be performed successfully by emergency physicians with few major immediate adverse events.

COMMENTARY
Although RSI became the standard of care in Level I trauma centers and community EDs, many academic training programs faced interdepartmental resistance to the use of paralytics in the ED. This study observed high success rates with few major immediate adverse outcomes in an urban, tertiary academic ED (even using midazolam as an induction agent) and contributed to breaking down these historical impediments to use, and training, of RSI in EM. Initial criticisms noted that these findings were limited to a single ED, but similar results and larger surveys at numerous other academic EDs have subsequently supported the generalizability of this work. Similar to many other studies of emergency airway management, readers should note that data was collected by nurses and residents during or after intubations. This may introduce information bias. These results firmly established the importance of RSI training for emergency medicine residents, thus securing RSI for airway management as an essential skill for the emergency physician.

Question
Can rapid sequence intubation (RSI) be performed successfully and safely by emergency medicine residents?

Answer
Yes, emergency medicine trainees demonstrate high rates of successful intubation using RSI with few major adverse events.

CHAPTER 11
HEMOGLOBIN DESATURATION AFTER SUCCINYLCHOLINE

Hemoglobin Desaturation After Succinylcholine-induced Apnea: A Study of the Recovery of Spontaneous Ventilation in Healthy Volunteers
Heier T, Feiner JR, Lin J, et al. *Anesthesiology.* 2001;94(5):754–759

BACKGROUND
Rapid sequence intubation (RSI) is now well established as a safe method for airway management in the ED. Succinylcholine is the most commonly used neuromuscular blocker during RSI because of its rapid onset and relatively short duration of action. Because of these properties, there was an anecdotal belief that patients would recover spontaneous breathing prior to significant desaturation. It was suggested that this anecdotal confidence led to an underestimation of the risks of succinylcholine-induced apnea.

OBJECTIVES
To determine whether healthy volunteers given succinylcholine in a controlled setting recover spontaneous respiratory function rapidly enough to prevent significant hemoglobin desaturation.

METHODS
Observational study in the anesthesia department of a single academic institution in 2000.

Participants
Twelve healthy volunteers, 18 to 45 years old. Select exclusion criteria: BMI >30, Mallampati score of 2 to 4, known allergy to thiopental or succinylcholine, family history of anesthesia-related complication, or drug or alcohol use.

Intervention
Participants were placed on cardiopulmonary monitoring including continuous pulse oximetry. After a period of preoxygenation with a nonrebreather to an end-tidal oxygen concentration of 90%, participants were induced with 5 mg/kg of thiopental and then given 1 mg/kg succinylcholine. Administration of supplemental oxygen, airway maneuvers, or assisted ventilation occurred only if patient's oxygen saturation fell below 80%.

Outcomes
The primary outcome was time from succinylcholine administration to recovery, indicated by (1) spontaneous respiration, (2) eye opening, and (3) hand squeeze. Secondary outcomes included the difference in apnea time between those with and without significant desaturation (SaO_2 >95% vs. <80%) and correlation of apnea duration with lowest SaO_2.

KEY RESULTS
- SaO_2 decreased below 95% in 50% (6/12) of participants and fell below 80% in 33% (4/12) requiring airway maneuvers and assisted ventilation.
- Apnea duration differed significantly in those with SaO_2 <80% compared to those without desaturation (7 ± 0.4 vs. 4.1 ± 0.3 min).
- A significant correlation was observed between lowest SaO_2 and duration of apnea ($R^2 = 0.78$).
- Mean recovery times were 5.2, 5.7, and 7.7 minutes for spontaneous respirations, eye opening, and hand squeeze, respectively.

STUDY CONCLUSIONS
Return of spontaneous respirations after succinylcholine may not occur quickly enough to prevent significant hemoglobin desaturation in patients without assisted ventilation.

COMMENTARY
This study of preoxygenated, healthy volunteers given a short-acting induction agent followed by succinylcholine demonstrated that prolonged apnea occurs in a substantial percentage of patients, and frequently results in significant oxygen desaturation. The period of "safe apnea," or the amount of time after succinylcholine administration during RSI in a sufficiently preoxygenated, healthy patient was approximately 5 minutes. If the airway cannot be secured during that time, airway maneuvers such as chin-lift/jaw-thrust or use of an oral airway and assisted ventilation should be initiated. It should be noted, however, that this study was conducted in young, healthy, nonobese subjects with at least 3 minutes of preoxygenation to an end-tidal oxygen saturation >90%. Given that intubations in the ED occur under less-than-ideal conditions in patients in extremis with multiple comorbidities, the true "safe apnea" period is likely far less than 5 minutes and may not exist for some. The variable response to thiopental is also a confounding factor. This study, however, debunked an important myth and reiterates the importance of preoxygenation when possible.

Question
Will patients given succinylcholine for rapid sequence intubation recover spontaneous ventilation prior to significant oxyhemoglobin desaturation?

Answer
No, emergency care providers should anticipate a significant desaturation in a substantial portion of patients given the short-acting paralytic.

CHAPTER 12
LARYNGEAL VIEW IMPROVEMENT IN LARYNGOSCOPY

Laryngeal View During Laryngoscopy: A Randomized Trial Comparing Cricoid Pressure, Back-Upward-Rightward Pressure, and Bimanual Laryngoscopy
Levitan RM, Kinkle WC, Levin WJ, et al. *Ann Emerg Med.* 2006;47(6):548–555

BACKGROUND
Endotracheal intubation is a complex, dynamic process, and the ability to view the larynx significantly impacts success rates. Various forms of external manipulation of the neck soft tissues have been taught to optimize laryngeal view during direct laryngoscopy. At the time of this study, results from prior, small studies led to significant controversy about which method most improved, or worsened, laryngeal exposure during intubation.

OBJECTIVES
To determine whether cricoid pressure, backward-upward-rightward pressure (BURP), or bimanual laryngoscopy best optimize laryngeal view compared to no external neck manipulation during direct laryngoscopy.

METHODS
Randomized intervention during 2-day, emergency airway cadaver-based workshops at a single academic department of EM in the United States.

Participants
Convenience sample of 104 clinicians: 89 EM attendings, 6 non-EM attendings, 6 PGY3 or PGY4 EM residents, 2 paramedics, and 1 physician assistant.

Intervention
After attempting intubation without external manipulation, using the same curved blade, each participant performed each of the following maneuvers in a randomly assigned sequence on the same cadaver: Sellick maneuver (cricoid pressure by an assistant), BURP (backward-upward-rightward pressure of thyroid cartilage by an assistant), and bimanual laryngeal manipulation (simultaneous visualization of the larynx and manipulation of the thyroid cartilage by the operator to optimize view with subsequent pressure by the assistant). The same assistant was used for each technique. Cadavers were fresh, nonformalin-fixed and arterially flushed with isopropyl alcohol to maintain tissue turgor.

Outcomes
Participants graded the view obtained after each method using the percentage of glottis opening visualized from 0% to 100%: 0% represented no visualization of the glottic opening and 100% indicated complete visualization. Based on prior work, a percentage change of 25% was considered to be clinically significant.

KEY RESULTS
- The mean improvement in view was 29% for bimanual, 25% for cricoid pressure, and 26% for BURP.
- 1,530 sets of comparative laryngoscopies were performed, 73% (1,118) of which had less than complete glottis visualization without neck manipulation.
- If the glottic opening was *not visualized* on initial attempt (n = 96), bimanual manipulation improved the view in 86% compared to 48% and 51% cricoid and BURP, respectively.
- If glottic opening was *visualized*, but with a suboptimal initial view, bimanual manipulation improved the view in 89% compared to 52% and 54% for cricoid and BURP, respectively.
- Cricoid pressure and BURP *worsened* views during attempts where the operator was able to visualize at least some of the glottic opening (n = 1,022) in 48% and 46% compared to only 11% for bimanual manipulation.

STUDY CONCLUSIONS
The percentage of glottic opening visualized varied significantly depending on the method of external manipulation used during curved-blade, direct laryngoscopy. Bimanual laryngoscopy provided the best views compared to BURP and cricoid pressure; the latter two more frequently and significantly worsened views.

COMMENTARY
The Sellick and BURP techniques of external neck soft tissue manipulation, which originated from anecdote and observational studies in the anesthesia literature, had been traditionally taught to EM residents for improving glottic views during direct laryngoscopy. This randomized study was the first to compare three methods of external laryngeal manipulation and demonstrated that bimanual manipulation provided significantly better glottic views, and did so more frequently. Importantly, the BURP and Sellick maneuvers worsened views almost as frequently as they improved them. Notably, this study did not look at rates of successful intubation. Furthermore this is a cadaver study, done under controlled conditions during an airway management course with primarily attending EM physicians. Despite these limitations, the finding that cricoid pressure and BURP did not improve, and often worsened, laryngeal views prompted a trend away from use of these maneuvers in the ED.

Question
Does the method of external neck manipulation significantly improve the quality of laryngeal view during intubation?

Answer
Selectively, bimanual manipulation more frequently improved glottic views; however, BURP and cricoid pressure were equally likely to improve or worsen views during direct laryngoscopy.

SECTION 3
ALLERGY

Christina Wilson ■ Brock Daniels

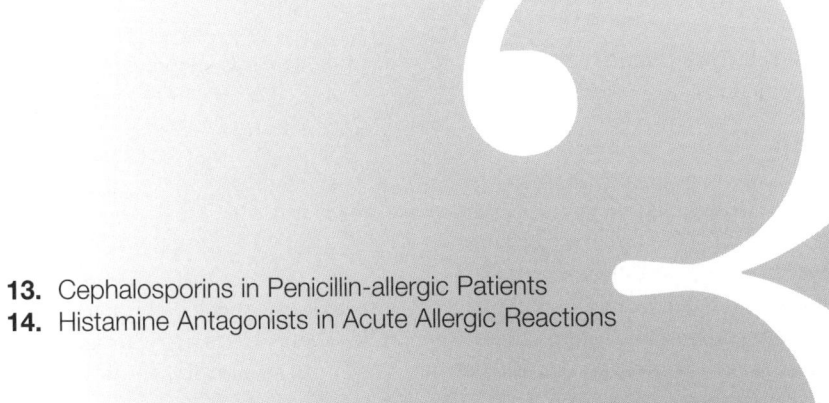

13. Cephalosporins in Penicillin-allergic Patients
14. Histamine Antagonists in Acute Allergic Reactions

CHAPTER 13
CEPHALOSPORINS IN PENICILLIN-ALLERGIC PATIENTS

Cross-reactivity and Tolerability of Cephalosporins in Patients with Immediate Hypersensitivity to Penicillins
Romano A, Guéant-Rodriguez RM, Viola M, et al. *Ann Intern Med.* 2004;141(1):16–22

BACKGROUND
Penicillins and first-generation beta-lactams are among the most commonly prescribed antibiotics, and frequently cited as a common cause of severe allergic reactions. Neither patient-reported history, nor penicillin skin tests reliably predict allergic reactions in patients with a history of penicillin allergy, and little consensus existed regarding whether administration of cephalosporins to such patients is safe. Inappropriate use may result in anaphylaxis while underuse when cephalosporins are indicated may result in increased cost, reduced effectiveness, or increased antimicrobial resistance. At the time of this study, estimates of sensitization to cephalosporins in patients with documented IgE-mediated hypersensitivity to penicillins varied.

OBJECTIVES
To evaluate the cross-reactivity in patients with documented IgE-mediated hypersensitivity to penicillins.

METHODS
Prospective cohort enrolled from an outpatient population followed at two allergy units in Italy between 1995 and 2003.

Participants
One hundred and twenty-eight patients with anaphylactic shock (81) or urticaria (47) and confirmation of IgE-mediated penicillin allergy by skin testing. Select exclusion criteria: Pregnancy, beta-blocker use or severe respiratory, cardiovascular, or renal compromise.

Intervention
Skin testing for cephalosporin sensitization was performed using reagents for first-generation, second-generation, and third-generation cephalosporins. Consenting patients with negative skin tests for second- and third-generation cephalosporins were administered test doses of PO cefuroxime and IM ceftriaxone.

Outcomes
The primary study outcome was proportion of positive skin tests for first-, second-, and third-generation cephalosporins. Secondary outcome included tolerability of cefuroxime and ceftriaxone in patients with negative cephalosporin skin tests.

KEY RESULTS
- 10.9% (14) of patients with confirmed penicillin allergy had positive skin tests indicating reaction to cephalosporins.
- All of the patients (94 with a negative cephalosporin skin test as well as 7 with a positive skin test who agreed to proceed) challenged with PO cefuroxime and IM ceftriaxone tolerated them well.

STUDY CONCLUSIONS
Cephalosporins should be avoided in patients with a history of IgE-mediated hypersensitivity with positive penicillin skin tests, as the cross-reactivity approaches 11%. In such patients with a therapeutic requirement for cephalosporins, cephalosporin-specific skin tests should be performed to assess tolerability.

COMMENTARY
Early studies using first-generation cephalosporins suggested high, but variable, rates of cross-reactivity in patients with a history of penicillin allergy. Results of cephalosporin skin tests suggest sensitization in 11%, confirming the need to avoid cephalosporins in patients with severe, immediate hypersensitivity reactions to penicillins. It should be noted, however, that two-thirds of those with positive skin tests tested positive for first- and older second-generation cephalosporins not currently used in the United States. Among those penicillin-allergic patients with negative cephalosporin skin tests, all tolerated oral cefuroxime and IM ceftriaxone. As cephalosporin formulations have evolved in an era of broader drug safety surveillance, recent studies suggest that the true incidence of significant cephalosporin cross-reactivity is closer to 1% to 2% in those with confirmed penicillin allergy.

Question
Can cephalosporins be used safely in patients with an allergy to penicillin?

Answer
Selectively, while 10% of patients with a history of a penicillin allergy had positive skin tests when exposed to cephalosporins, none experienced anaphylaxis. The administration of later generation cephalosporins may be even safer.

CHAPTER 14: HISTAMINE ANTAGONISTS IN ACUTE ALLERGIC REACTION

Improved Outcomes in Patients with Acute Allergic Syndromes who are Treated with Combined H1 and H2 Antagonists

Lin RY, Curry A, Pesola GR, et al. *Ann Emerg Med.* 2000;36(5):462–468

BACKGROUND

H_2-receptor antagonists were introduced as antacid medications in the late 1970s. Physicians started using H_2-blockers to treat allergic reactions, based on the theoretical benefit of increased histamine blockade. Prior to this study, there had been evaluation of H_2 blockade in *preventing* allergic reactions, but only one study had examined outcomes in treating patients with acute allergic reaction.

OBJECTIVES

To determine whether combined therapy with H_1 and H_2 antihistamines results in improved outcomes in patients with acute allergic symptoms.

METHODS

Randomized, double-blind, placebo-controlled trial conducted in a single urban academic ED between 1998 and 1999.

Patients

Ninety-one adult patients with acute urticaria, angioedema, stridor, or pruritic rash after ingested food, contact with latex or ingested, inhaled, or injected drug.

Intervention Evaluated

Patients were treated either with 50-mg IV diphenhydramine and 50-mg IV ranitidine, or with 50-mg IV diphenhydramine and IV saline solution.

Outcomes

Primary outcomes were resolution of urticaria, angioedema, or erythema at 2 hours after treatment. Secondary outcomes were area of cutaneous involvement, heart rate, blood pressure, respiratory status, and symptom score at baseline, 1 hour, and 2 hours after treatment.

KEY RESULTS

- At 2 hours post-treatment, 91.7% of patients treated with H_1 and H_2 blockade were urticaria-free compared to 73.8% in those treated with H_1 blockade and placebo.
- Odds ratio of 4.7 ($p = 0.03$) in favor of combination treatment for resolution of urticaria.
- There was no significant difference between the two groups with respect to skin erythema, angioedema, blood pressure, or overall symptoms.

STUDY CONCLUSIONS

Treatment with diphenhydramine plus ranitidine results in higher rates of urticaria resolution than treatment with diphenhydramine alone, supporting the recommendation to use combined histamine blockade in acute allergic reaction.

> **COMMENTARY**
>
> This randomized, controlled trial generally supports the now-routine use of H_2-blockers in treatment of acute allergic reaction. Limitations include lack of benefit in angioedema, which can have differing pathophysiology, and inability to extrapolate for more severe reaction and anaphylaxis as only 12 patients had respiratory symptoms and only 2 patients had hypotension. Of note, the Cochrane Skin Group subsequently published a review (*Histamine H_2-receptor antagonists for urticaria*, March 2012) reviewing all available data and concluded that the evidence was "weak and unreliable" and that current evidence "does not allow confident decision making" regarding the use of combined antihistamine therapy.

Question

Does combination treatment with H_1- and H_2-blockers improve outcomes in patients presenting to the ED with acute allergic reactions?

Answer

Yes, combination therapy with H_1- and H_2-blockers shows more improvement in urticarial symptoms; however, it does not decrease other symptoms of anaphylaxis when compared to H_1-blockers alone.

SECTION 4

CARDIOLOGY

Kenneth Bernard ■ Stephanie E. Burgos ■ Peter B. Pruitt
Harman S. Gill ■ Joshua M. Keegan

15. TIMI Risk Score for ACS
16. Acute MI Without Chest Pain
17. Missed ACS in the ED
18. Troponins in Chest Pain
19. Beta-Blockers in Acute MI: The COMMIT Trial
20. Aspirin in Acute MI: The ISIS-2 Trial
21. Heparinizing Unstable Angina
22. Low-Molecular-Weight Heparin in Unstable Angina
23. tPA in Acute MI: The Gusto Trial
24. PCI vs. Lytics in Acute MI: The Gusto IIB Trial
25. PCI Timing in ACS
26. Delaying Defibrillation for CPR in Cardiac Arrest
27. Therapeutic Hypothermia in Cardiac Arrest
28. CPR Quality in Out-of-Hospital Cardiac Arrest
29. Chest Compression Only CPR
30. Amiodarone in Ventricular Fibrillation
31. Epinephrine in Cardiac Arrest
32. tPA in PEA Cardiac Arrest
33. Vasopressin vs. Epinephrine for Cardiac Arrest
34. Pill-in-the-Pocket Approach for Atrial Fibrillation
35. Rhythm Control in Atrial Fibrillation: The Affirm Trial
36. Risk of Stroke in Atrial Fibrillation Cardioversion

CHAPTER 15 TIMI RISK SCORE FOR ACS

The TIMI Risk Score for Unstable Angina/Non-ST Elevation MI: A Method for Prognostication and Therapeutic Decision Making
Antman EM, Cohen M, Bernink PJ, et al. *JAMA.* 2000;284(7):835–842

BACKGROUND
Patients presenting to the ED with unstable angina (UA) or non-ST–segment elevation myocardial infarction (NSTEMI) represent a heterogenous population with varying risk of adverse outcomes such as death and major adverse cardiac events. Prior to this study risk stratification was based on clinical judgment without objective criteria.

OBJECTIVES
This study aimed to develop a simple, generalizable risk stratification tool for evaluation of patients with UA/NSTEMI as well as to identify patients with different risk profiles and responses to treatments for UA/NSTEMI.

METHODS
Observational analysis of two previously conducted randomized controlled trials.

Patients
7,081 patients with UA/NSTEMI from the efficacy and safety of subcutaneous enoxaparin in non-Q–wave coronary events (ESSENCE) and thrombolysis in myocardial infarction (TIMI) 11B trials. These were double-blinded, placebo-controlled trials that randomly assigned patients to receive enoxaparin or unfractionated heparin.

Intervention Evaluated
Independent risk predictor variables were selected and using multivariate logistic regression. Statistically significant predictors were selected to create the TIMI risk score. The risk score was then validated in three cohorts of patients from different testing arms of the above trials.

Outcomes
The primary outcome was a composite of all-cause mortality, new or recurrent MI, or severe recurrent ischemia requiring urgent revascularization 14 days after randomization. Also, the study sought to evaluate differences in response to therapeutic interventions by testing for an interaction between TIMI risk score and treatment options.

KEY RESULTS
- Seven identified TIMI risk score predictor variables:
  1. Age 65 years or older
  2. At least three risk factors for coronary artery disease

3. Prior coronary stenosis of 50% or more
4. ST-segment deviation on electrocardiogram at presentation
5. At least two anginal events in prior 24 hours
6. Use of aspirin in prior 7 days
7. Elevated serum cardiac markers
- Adverse event rates increased as the TIMI risk score increased. Patients with a TIMI risk score of 0 or 1 had a 4.7% rate of the composite outcome, while patients with a score of 6 or 7 had a 40.9% event rate.
- The pattern of increasing event rates with increasing TIMI risk score was confirmed in all three validation groups.
- Patients with higher TIMI risk scores had better outcomes when treated with enoxaparin compared to those treated with unfractionated heparin.

STUDY CONCLUSIONS

In patients with UA/NSTEMI, the TIMI risk score is a simple prognostication scheme that categorizes a patient's risk of death and ischemic events in the first 14 days after presentation to the ED and provides a basis for therapeutic decision making.

COMMENTARY

Risk stratification models identify patients at high risk of adverse outcomes for whom there is a unique need for closer monitoring, specialty consultation, and potential interventions. The TIMI risk score is a clinical prediction rule that can be quickly and easily applied based on a patient's history alone. It has a modest accuracy with C statistic of 0.63 of predicting the composite endpoint and 0.72 to 0.78 of predicting mortality. The TIMI risk score has been a practice-changing clinical decision tool that has aided in the creation of ED chest pain protocols and pathways for effective and efficient evaluations of a very common ED complaint. Although well derived and validated, even at a score of 0 or 1 there was a nearly 5% incidence of adverse events, which means that at this time a very low TIMI risk score alone is not sufficient to discharge low-risk patients without further testing or follow-up.

Question

Can the TIMI risk score be used in ED patients with UA/NSTEMI to predict short-term adverse outcomes including death?

Answer

Yes, the TIMI risk score is a simple tool that allows emergency physicians to predict outcomes in ED patients with UA/NSTEMI, but even 5% of patients in the lowest risk group experienced adverse outcomes within 14 days.[1]

Reference

1. Anderson JL, Adams CD, Antman EM; ACC/AHA 2007 guidelines for the management of patients with unstable angina/non ST-elevation myocardial infarction: a report of the American College of Cardiology/American Heart Association Task Force on Practice Guidelines (Writing Committee to Revise the 2002 Guidelines for the Management of Patients With Unstable Angina/Non ST-Elevation Myocardial Infarction). *J Am Coll Cardiol.* 2007;50:e1–e157.

CHAPTER 16: ACUTE MI WITHOUT CHEST PAIN

Prevalence, Clinical Characteristics, and Mortality Among Patients with Myocardial Infarction Presenting Without Chest pain
Canto JG1, Shlipak MG, Rogers WJ, et al. *JAMA.* 2000;283(24):3223–3229

BACKGROUND
AMI is a primary cause of mortality in the United States, however 2% to 3% of the time this diagnosis is missed and patients are sent home. While patients most often present with chest pain, as the Pope et al.[1] study showed (see Chapter 16), presenting with an alternate chief complaint, such as shortness of breath, made it more likely that MI would be missed. This study sought to characterize the population of patients with MI who present without chest pain.

OBJECTIVES
To determine the frequency that patients with MI present without chest pain and to examine their clinical characteristics, subsequent management, and outcome.

METHODS
Prospective observational study using NRMI-2, a national registry designed to collect hospital data on patients admitted with an MI.

Participants
434,877 patients with confirmed MI by one of the following: (1) CK-MB or total CK greater than or equal to twice the upper limits of normal; (2) ischemic EKG changes; (3) other enzymes or autopsy findings indicating MI; (4) diagnosis code associated with MI.

Intervention Evaluated
Chest pain was defined as any symptom of chest discomfort or pressure, or arm, neck, or jaw pain. The chest pain variable was defined as the absence of chest pain before or during admission and may have included (but not limited to) dyspnea, nausea/vomiting, palpitations, syncope, or cardiac arrest.

Outcomes
The prevalence of an MI without chest pain and the clinical characteristics, treatment, and mortality among MI patients without chest pain vs. those with chest pain.

KEY RESULTS
- 33% of patients with MI presented without chest pain. Women and patients greater than 75 years of age were more likely to present without chest pain.

- Six major risk factors of MI presenting without chest pain were identified: Female, nonwhite, diabetes, hypertension, prior heart failure, and stroke.
- EKG was obtained much later in patients presenting with MI without chest pain (31.8 vs. 15.6 minutes).
- Patients without chest pain were less likely to receive aspirin, heparin, or beta-blockers within the first 24 hours. They were also less likely to be treated with reperfusion therapy.
- Patients who had an MI with no chest pain had a more than twofold increased risk of inhospital death when compared to those who presented with chest pain (23.3% vs. 9.3%).

STUDY CONCLUSIONS

Over one-third of patients with acute MI present without chest pain, and these patients are at increased risk for delays in seeking medical attention, less aggressive treatments, and inhospital mortality.

COMMENTARY

As the leading cause of death in the United States, improving the diagnosis and treatment of acute MI has been the foundation of decades of research and clinical discovery. This study highlights the importance of recognizing that patients with acute MI often do not have chest pain, and that atypical presentations can be more challenging to diagnose and subsequently result in worse outcomes. Because of these findings, broad protocols have been implemented around EKG acquisition for patients over the age of 50 years with symptoms such as shortness of breath, syncope, and abdominal pain and there have been initiatives focusing on educating providers about atypical presentations. This study also paved the way for patient education and awareness campaigns by the American Heart Association. These were designed to encourage both women and patients with diabetes, who may have atypical presentation, to seek care.

Question

How many patients with acute MI present without chest pain? Do patients with acute MI without chest pain have worse outcomes?

Answer

Yes, 1/3 of patients with acute MI present without chest pain, and these patients have an increased risk of misdiagnosis, treatment delay, and mortality.

Reference

1. Pope JH, Aufderheide TP, Ruthazer R, et al. Missed diagnoses of acute cardiac ischemia in the emergency department. *N Engl J Med.* 2000;342(16):1163–1170.

CHAPTER 17   MISSED ACS IN THE ED

Missed Diagnoses of Acute Cardiac Ischemia in the Emergency Department
Pope J, Aufderheide TP, Ruthazer R, et al. *N Engl J Med.* 2000;342(16):1163–1170

BACKGROUND
Chest pain is one of the leading chief complaints in the ED and acute coronary syndrome (ACS) is a complicated clinical diagnosis with significant medicolegal implications. The authors estimate that at the time of the study there were 1.1 million myocardial infarctions (MIs) annually with around 11,000 missed in the United States. However, there was no data on missed cases of unstable angina (UA). ACS frequently presents atypically and in patients without significant risk factors. Prior to this study there was very little information about how often emergency physicians missed MI and what the resulting consequences were.

OBJECTIVES
To evaluate how frequently ED providers failed to hospitalize patients ultimately diagnosed with ACS, including both MI and UA, and how this misdiagnosis affected mortality.

METHODS
Prospective study conducted in 10 academic and community EDs over 7 months in 1993.

Participants
10,689 patients, >30 years old, with symptoms that could represent acute ischemia (e.g., chest pain, shortness of breath, epigastric pain).

Interventions
Patient data including demographics, symptoms/examination findings, EKGs and CK-MB levels were collected at presentation, 48 to 72 hours and then at 30 days (no CK-MB at 30 days). Follow-up data was obtained on 99% of patients.

Outcomes
Primary outcomes were number of patients with MI or UA who were missed. Secondary outcomes included 30-day mortality and the clinical characteristics of those patients.

KEY RESULTS
- 2.1% of patients with MI and 2.3% of patients with UA were not hospitalized.
- Emergency physicians accurately interpreted EKGs: Only 2 of the 19 EKGs of patients with missed MI were subsequently read by a cardiologist as showing MI and only 3 of the 19 EKGs of patients with missed UA were subsequently read by a cardiologist showing UA.

- Patients with ischemia who were not hospitalized were more likely to be nonwhite and to present with the chief complaint of shortness of breath.
- The unadjusted 30-day mortality for patients with acute MI who were discharged was 10.5% compared to 9.7% for those who were admitted. However, when they adjusted for predicted 30-day mortality, they found that the relative risk of not being admitted was 1.9.

STUDY CONCLUSIONS

The rate of missed MI in the ED is relatively low (2.1%) but leads to increased mortality. Women are more likely to get discharged with ACS, as are African Americans and those who present primarily complaining of shortness of breath.

COMMENTARY

Prior to this paper, there was significant concern about litigation for missed MI but little research on the subject; this paper addressed this knowledge gap. Because of its size and power, this paper's findings (that missed MI increases mortality) help lay the foundation for today's practice of an aggressive diagnostic strategy in the ED for ACS. This paper led to broad changes in the EM community, including the adoption of chest pain units and rapid, sensitive troponin assays to decrease the ACS miss rate. This paper also exposed the role of atypical presentations and social factors such as age, race, and gender. The 4% absolute rate of missed AMI found in this study should now be interpreted with some caution as the advances in emergency cardiac care, national public awareness campaigns, and prevention efforts have likely reduced this figure considerably.

Question
Are there factors that make a patient more likely to have their acute MI missed in the ED?

Answer
Yes, demographic factors including African American race and female gender as well as clinical factors such as a chief complaint of shortness of breath all increase the likelihood that a patient will be discharged from the ED with a missed diagnosis of acute MI.

CHAPTER 18 TROPONINS IN CHEST PAIN

Emergency Room Triage of Patients with Acute Chest Pain by Means of Rapid Testing for Cardiac Troponin T or Troponin I
Hamm CW, Goldmann BU, Heeschen C, et al. *N Engl J Med.* 1997;337:1648–1653

BACKGROUND
Acute chest pain is one of the most common reasons for ED presentation and has been the subject of decades of research to identify efficient approaches to diagnosing acute MI. As chest pain can be caused by a spectrum of disease from benign muscular strain to fatal acute coronary syndrome (ACS), it is a diagnostic challenge with medicolegal risk, morbidity, and mortality. Prior to this study patients with indeterminate EKGs occupied expensive beds in coronary care units while CK and CK-MB were measured over time, but these markers were nonspecific and had questionable prognostic value and poor specificity.

OBJECTIVES
To compare the efficacy of cardiac biomarkers—troponins T and I—in the ED evaluation and treatment of acute chest pain.

METHODS
A prospective trial at the University Hospital in Hamburg, Germany between June 1994 and March 1996.

Patients
Seven hundred and seventy-three consecutive patients of all ages who had acute anterior, precordial or left-sided chest pain lasting 12 hours or less unexplained by obvious local trauma and/or abnormalities on chest x-ray. Select exclusion criteria: ST segment elevations or documented acute MI during the preceding 2 weeks.

Intervention
Twelve-lead EKG, troponin T and troponin I biomarkers were obtained within 15 minutes of arrival and 4 hours later. Patients who presented less than 2 hours after the onset of chest pain had these tests performed for a third time 6 hours after the onset of pain.

Outcomes
Primary outcomes were death from cardiac causes and nonfatal acute MI during hospitalization (excluding the first 24 hours) or after discharge from the hospital, as shown by hospital records. Death from MI was counted only as a death from cardiac causes. All patients were followed until discharge from the hospital and for 30 days or by telephone or questionnaire to record cardiac events (97.2% had complete follow-up data).

KEY RESULTS
- Of 773 patients with chest pain, 47 had acute MI—44 (94%) had positive troponin T tests and 47 (100%) had positive troponin I tests.
- Of the remaining 726 patients, unstable angina was diagnosed in 315 patients. Of these, 22% (70) had at least one positive troponin T test and 36% (114) had at least one positive troponin I test.
- Seven patients had a positive troponin T but a negative troponin I—six of these patients had associated renal failure.
- Among 158 patients with ST segment depressions, 32% (51) had at least one positive troponin T test and 56% (88) had at least one positive troponin I test. Among 197 patients with T-wave inversions, 6% (12) had at least one positive troponin T test and 5% (9) had at least one positive troponin I test.
- During 30 days of follow-up, there were 20 deaths and 14 nonfatal MIs. The event rates in patients with negative tests were only 1.1% for troponin T and 0.3% with troponin I.

CONCLUSIONS
Bedside tests for cardiac-specific biomarkers have high sensitivity for early detection of acute MI and ACS. In conjunction with an appropriate history and physical examination, serial EKG evaluation, and appropriate aftercare, these tests can be used for rapid ED evaluation and discharge of patients.

COMMENTARY
The lack of sensitive and specific biomarker assays for the diagnosis of acute MI had long precluded efficient diagnostic pathways for patients with chest pain. This study was the first large, prospective study to collect detailed patient histories as well as comparative data between troponin T and I, older biomarkers and associated EKG findings. The primary finding of remarkably high sensitivity for the diagnosis of AMI and prediction of 30-day events demonstrated the utility of short-term serial troponins in patients with chest pain. These findings revolutionized chest pain care in the ED by encouraging the development of accelerated diagnostic protocols and the eventual transition away from older nonspecific biomarkers to troponin assays. The study's impressive 97.2% follow-up rate is a strength, but readers should remember that serial troponins represent only a portion of the evaluation for ACS in patients with chest pain. Select patients still require provocative testing alongside these highly sensitive biomarkers.

Question
Does troponin T and I testing in the ED impact the evaluation of patients with acute chest pain?

Answer
Yes, as a result of very high sensitivity and specificity, troponin assays, when combined with history, physical examination, and serial EKGs, can rapidly diagnose AMIs and also identify low-risk patients suitable for accelerated discharge.

CHAPTER 19
BETA-BLOCKERS IN ACUTE MI: THE COMMIT TRIAL

Early Intravenous then Oral Metoprolol in 45,852 Patients with Acute Myocardial Infarction: Randomized Placebo-controlled Trial
Chen ZM, Pan HC, Chen YP, et al. *Lancet.* 2005;366(9497):1622–1632

BACKGROUND
Acute myocardial infarction (MI) is the leading cause of death in the United States, with approximately 450,000 people dying from acute MI each year. Although beta-blockers have known benefit in congestive heart failure (CHF), cardiac dysrhythmias, and Hypertension (HTN), their use in the setting of AMI was poorly understood. A number of randomized trials had shown benefit, but almost all were completed before the routine use of fibrinolytic and antiplatelet therapies, and the trials primarily studied low-risk patients. Since fibrinolytic therapy had shown a slight increase in mortality in the first days after symptom onset due to dysrhythmias and cardiac rupture, it was thought that beta-blockers could help suppress these adverse events and improve mortality if used in addition to standard therapy for acute MI.

OBJECTIVES
To assess the risks and benefits associated with the use of early beta-blocker therapy in acute MI.

METHODS
Randomized, multicenter placebo-controlled trial conducted at 1,250 hospitals in China.

Patients
45,852 patients with acute MI who presented within 24 hours of symptom onset. Select exclusion criteria: PCI or contraindications to study treatment as determined by the responsible physician.

Intervention Evaluated
Metoprolol or placebo, 5 mg IV given immediately, and every 2 to 3 minutes for up to three doses for HR >50 bpm and SBP >90 mm Hg followed by an uptitrating oral metoprolol for 4 weeks.

Outcomes
The primary outcome was a composite of death, reinfarction, or cardiac arrest. Secondary outcomes included death from any cause during the first 28 days. Secondary endpoints were reinfarction, ventricular fibrillation, other cardiac arrest, and cardiogenic shock.

KEY RESULTS
- No significant difference in coprimary outcomes of death, reinfarction, cardiac arrest (9.4% vs. 9.9%), and death from all causes (7.7% vs. 7.8%).
- The secondary outcomes showed reduction in reinfarction in the treatment group (2% vs. 2.5%) and a reduction of ventricular fibrillation in the treatment group (2.5% vs. 3%).
- Increase in the incidence of cardiogenic shock in the treatment group (5% vs. 3.9%).

STUDY CONCLUSIONS
There is no significant benefit to the use of early beta-blocker therapy as measured by death, reinfarction, or cardiac arrest.

COMMENTARY
This pivotal study debunked the potentially dangerous practice of routinely administering early beta-blocker therapy to patients with acute MI—a practice which had become ubiquitous prior to this study and was driven by the desire to seek out any treatment that could potentially impact this leading cause of death. This study demonstrated that early use of beta-blocker therapy not only had little benefit in the acute management, but in fact carried with it a risk of cardiogenic shock, which came as a great surprise to many. Although the results of this study dramatically changed practice, it should be noted that this was prior to the widespread use of antiplatelet therapy and availability of early percutaneous coronary intervention.

Question
Should beta-blockers routinely be given to patients who present with acute MI?

Answer
No, the routine use of IV beta-blockers in the ED for acute MI may increase the risk of cardiogenic shock. They should, therefore, be reserved for hemodynamically stable patients with elevated blood pressures to reduce the risk of reinfarction and ventricular fibrillation.

CHAPTER 20
ASPIRIN IN ACUTE MI: THE ISIS-2 TRIAL

Randomized Trial of Intravenous Streptokinase, Oral Aspirin, Both, or Neither Among 17,187 Cases of Suspected Acute Myocardial Infarction: ISIS-2. ISIS-2 (Second International Study of Infarct Survival) Collaborative Group

Lancet. 1988;332(8607):349–360

BACKGROUND

At the time of this study, work had been done showing that fibrinolysis reduced mortality by about 25% in the acute setting and that there was a benefit to aspirin in those with a history of previous MI, but those studies lacked power to be definitive. There was a need to assess whether aspirin could help reduce reinfarction following fibrinolytic therapy given that this was a cause of acute MI mortality and morbidity.

OBJECTIVE

To assess the separate and combined effects of IV streptokinase and oral aspirin in patients with acute MI.

METHODS

Randomized controlled trial at 417 hospitals in 16 countries.

Patients

17,187 patients who presented within 24 hours of onset of suspected acute MI. Select exclusion criteria: History of stroke, GI bleed, or ulcer.

Intervention Evaluated

Patients were randomized to one of four treatment groups: (1) a 1-hour IV infusion of 1.5 million units of streptokinase; (2) 1 month of 160 mg/day aspirin; (3) both active treatments; or (4) neither.

Outcomes

Effect on vascular and all-cause mortality in the first 5 weeks after treatment.

KEY RESULTS
- Those who received streptokinase had a 25% reduction in the odds of death when compared to the placebo group.
- Within this group, the greatest reduction in death was found in those given streptokinase at 0 to 4 hours, however, there was still a significant reduction for those given it within 4 to 24 hours.
- Significant increase (0.1%) of confirmed cerebral hemorrhage was found with streptokinase usage in comparison to placebo.

- Patients who received aspirin had a 23% reduction in the odds of death at 5 weeks when compared to those that received placebo.
- Patients who received the combination of streptokinase and aspirin had a 42% reduced mortality at 5 weeks when compared to those who received placebo.
- One month of low-dose aspirin started in the acute period after an MI would avoid 25 deaths and 10 to 15 nonfatal reinfarctions or strokes.

STUDY CONCLUSIONS

Both fibrinolytic therapy and antiplatelet therapy (in isolation and together) significantly reduces death and reinfarction for patients with an acute MI.

COMMENTARY

ISIS-2 is one of the pioneering studies in thrombolysis for acute MI. This study was one of the pivotal studies to demonstrate the combined efficacy of fibrinolytics and antiplatelet therapy, in acute MI. Prior to this there were few studies looking at medical therapies for acute MI along with limited PCI options. This study was unique in that it was a large randomized trial that proved the combination of aspirin and fibrinolytics significantly reduces mortality in acute MI. It should be noted that the relative reduction in mortality from early aspirin therapy was almost equal to that of thrombolysis leading to national efforts to ensure that all patients with acute MI receive aspirin from prehospital providers or in the ED. Also, the marked mortality benefit found for streptokinase in this study triggered the development of newer generation fibrinolytics that continue to save lives in areas without access to PCI.

Question

Does aspirin improve outcomes in patients with a STEMI? What about aspirin combined with fibrinolytics?

Answer

Yes, aspirin reduces mortality in STEMI, and the combination of aspirin with fibrinolysis reduces mortality even more.

CHAPTER 21

HEPARINIZING UNSTABLE ANGINA

Adding Heparin to Aspirin Reduces the Incidence of Myocardial Infarction and Death in Patients with Unstable Angina: A Meta-analysis
Oler A, Whooley MA, Oler J, et al. *JAMA*. 1996;276(10):811–815

BACKGROUND
Prospective studies had shown that 12% of patients hospitalized with unstable angina (UA) had an MI within 2 weeks with 1-year mortality ranging from 5% to 14% at the time of this study. Heparin had previously been shown to have benefit when used in patients with ST-elevation MI and during percutaneous coronary intervention, but prior randomized trials in the setting of UA had been unable to establish a definitive benefit of combination therapy regarding death or MI.

OBJECTIVES
To examine the effect on a composite endpoint of progression to MI or death in patients treated with heparin and aspirin compared to patients treated with aspirin alone.

METHODS
Meta-analysis of six studies conducted globally between the years 1966 and 1995.

Studies Included
Six randomized controlled trials, representing 1,353 patients, admitted with either UA or non–Q-wave MI.

Intervention Studied
Studies randomized patients to either aspirin alone or dual therapy of aspirin plus heparin.

Outcome
Primary outcome was the incidence of Q wave, ST-elevation or CK-MB-evidenced MI, or death during the treatment period (2 to 7 days). Secondary outcomes included recurrent pain, major bleeding, 12-week death or MI, and 12-week revascularization procedures.

KEY RESULTS
- The incidence of death or MI within the treatment period with dual therapy was 7.9% compared with 10.4% in the group treated with aspirin alone (relative risk of 0.67; $p = 0.06$).
- The 12-week incidence of death or MI was 12.4% in the dual therapy group compared with 13.8% with aspirin alone. No p-value was reported for this result.

- The same number of patients underwent revascularization (about 23.5%) in the dual therapy compared to the aspirin-alone group.
- 1.5% of patients in the dual therapy group developed major bleeding compared with 0.4% in the aspirin-alone group; however, this result was not statistically significant.

STUDY CONCLUSIONS

There was a 33% relative risk reduction for MI or death in patients with UA treated with dual therapy when compared to aspirin alone. This suggests that most patients with UA should be treated with dual therapy compared with aspirin alone.

COMMENTARY

While early research had demonstrated value in the use of heparin for ST Elevation MI (STEMI) and non-ST Elevation MI (NSTEMI), that work had not included patients with UA. This meta-analysis was able to aggregate several studies of heparinization that had not been able to achieve adequate power alone. The investigators were not able to differentiate between death and MI when assessing outcomes, however, they noted that in studies reporting death and MI distinctly, most MIs were nonfatal. This study showed a near-significant result favoring therapy with heparin in addition to aspirin when looking at a group of relatively homogenous studies; however, the study conclusions emphatically recommended heparinization for patients with UA. The most recent review of the literature offers no greater clarity: A 2010 Cochrane review[1] found that for patients with ACS, there was a decreased incidence of MI with heparin, but no change in mortality. The current clinical practice guidelines support the use of heparin in the setting of UA, which may be due to these modestly favorable findings amidst a paucity of other proven treatments, uncertain outcomes from this dynamic condition, and medicolegal concerns.

Question

Does heparin improve outcomes in ED patients with unstable angina?

Answer

Maybe, IV heparin has been shown to decrease the likelihood of death in several smaller studies; however, in a metaanalysis this effect did not reach the same degree of statistical certainty as most recommendations in clinical medicine.

Reference

1. Magee K, Campbell SG, Moher D, Rowe BH. Heparin versus placebo for acute coronary syndromes. *Cochrane Database of Systematic Reviews.* 2008, Issue 2. Art. No.: CD003462. DOI: 10.1002/14651858. CD003462.pub2.

CHAPTER 22: LOW-MOLECULAR-WEIGHT HEPARIN IN UNSTABLE ANGINA

Enoxaparin Prevents Death and Cardiac Ischemic Events in Unstable Angina/Non-Q-Wave Myocardial Infarction: Results of the Thrombolysis in Myocardial Infarction (TIMI) 11B Trial

Antman E, McCabe CH, Gurfinkel EP, et al. *Circulation.* 1999;100:1593–1601

BACKGROUND
At the time of this study, some work had shown that heparin, in addition to fibrinolytics, reduced mortality in acute coronary syndrom (ACS); however, this had been limited to studies looking at STEMI. Low-molecular-weight heparin (LMWH) had not been investigated in the treatment of ACS. This study tested the hypothesis that LMWH was superior to unfractioned heparin (UFH) in preventing death and cardiac ischemic events in unstable angina/non–Q-wave myocardial infarction, a recognized form of acute MI.

OBJECTIVES
To test the benefit of enoxaparin (LMWH) compared with the standard treatment of UFH in patients with unstable angina/non–Q-wave MI in reducing death and further cardiac ischemic events.

METHODS
Double-blinded randomized controlled trial in 200 centers across three countries.

Patients
3,910 patients with ischemic discomfort (greater than or equal to 5 minutes duration within 24 hours of presentation) and ST deviation or positive serum cardiac biomarkers. Select exclusion criteria: History of coronary artery bypass graft (CABG), planned revascularization within 24 hours, and an evolving Q-wave MI.

Intervention Evaluated
There were two treatment phases during the trial: (1) an acute phase which consisted of the initial hospitalization and (2) an outpatient phase that looked at benefit of enoxaparin for 35 days after discharge. Patients were randomized to one of two treatments: (1) UFH with bolus infusion for at least 3 days vs. (2) enoxaparin bolus followed by subcutaneous injection every 12 hours. All patients received both IV infusion and subcutaneous injections to keep the intervention double-blinded.

Outcomes
Primary end point was a composite of all-cause mortality, recurrent MI, or urgent revascularization. Secondary outcomes included the individual elements of the primary end point.

KEY RESULTS
- By 8 days, the primary end point occurred in 14.5% of patients in the UFH group and 12.4% of patients in the enoxaparin group; by 43 days, it occurred in 19.7% of UFH group and 17.3% of the enoxaparin group.
- At 48 hours there was a 23.4% risk reduction in the primary end point in the enoxaparin group as compared to the UFH group; by 8 days this number dropped to 14.6%.
- There was no difference in the rate of major hemorrhage in the two treatment groups during the acute phase and initial hospitalization.
- Major hemorrhage occurred in 1.5% of the group treated with placebo and 2.9% of the group treated with enoxaparin ($p = 0.021$) during the outpatient phase.

STUDY CONCLUSIONS
For the acute management of unstable angina/non–Q-wave MIs, enoxaparin is superior to UFH for reducing a composite of death and serious cardiac ischemic events.

COMMENTARY
Unstable angina falls into the spectrum of ACS and suggests that a patient is at high risk for a future MI. Prior to this study, the antithrombin of choice was UFH which requires routine laboratory checks to assess partial thromboplastin time (PTT). This study shows that enoxaparin is superior in the acute treatment phase of UA with a risk reduction of 23.8% within 48 hours and 14.6% within 8 days of the composite outcome in comparison to UFH. Given the risk reduction with enoxaparin in comparison to UFH and easier administration without laboratory tests to follow, overall costs are less using enoxaparin. Notably, at 8 days the main difference in outcomes was with respect to recurrent MI, whereas at 14 days and 43 days the difference found in the outcome was largely due to differences in the need for urgent revascularization. This study contributed to the knowledge base that has ultimately led to a change in practice, now favoring LMWH for UA.

Question
Is LMWH superior to unfractionated heparin for the treatment of acute MI?

Answer
Yes, in comparison to unfractionated heparin, enoxaparin reduces the likelihood of death or serious cardiovascular outcomes.

CHAPTER 23

tPA IN ACUTE MI: THE GUSTO TRIAL

An International Randomized Trial Comparing Four Thrombolytic Strategies for Acute Myocardial Infarction. The Gusto Investigators
N Engl J Med. 1993;329(10):673–682

BACKGROUND
Although the ISIS-2 showed a survival benefit for streptokinase in acute MI in 1988, there had been no subsequent studies confirming additional benefit with other fibrinolytic therapies for acute MI. There had been studies showing no difference in associated mortality between the use of streptokinase and the use of tissue plasminogen activator (tPA) in acute MI but no research into the timing of thrombolytics and the combination of thrombolytics with heparin.

OBJECTIVES
To compare the effects of four thrombolytic strategies on mortality: Streptokinase with subcutaneous heparin, streptokinase with IV heparin, accelerated tPA with IV heparin, and streptokinase with tPA and IV heparin.

METHODS
Randomized prospective trial in 1,081 hospitals in 15 countries between 1990 and 1993.

Patients
41,021 patients with AMI who presented between 20 minutes and 6 hours of symptom onset and with ischemic EKG changes. Select exclusion criteria: Previous stroke, active bleeding, prior treatment with streptokinase or anistreplase, recent trauma, or major surgery.

Intervention Evaluated
Patients were randomized to one of four IV thrombolytic strategies: (1) streptokinase bolus followed by subcutaneous heparin every 12 hours; (2) streptokinase bolus with IV heparin bolus followed by an IV heparin infusion; (3) accelerated tPA bolus and IV heparin bolus followed by an IV heparin infusion; (4) combination of tPA, streptokinase, and IV heparin.

Outcomes
The primary outcome was death from any cause at 30-day follow-up. Secondary outcomes included nonfatal stroke, nonfatal hemorrhagic stroke, and nonfatal disabling stroke within 30 days.

KEY RESULTS
- Fourteen percent relative reduction in mortality with accelerated tPA when compared with the two streptokinase regimens. No difference in mortality between the combination therapy and the two streptokinase monotherapies.

- Ten percent risk reduction with the use of accelerated tPA and the combination therapy, and a significant difference in 30-day mortality.
- tPA led to 10 additional lives saved per 1,000 patients treated when compared to the streptokinase regimens.
- There was a small excess of 2 per 1,000 strokes within the accelerated tPA group when compared to streptokinase, but there was a net advantage over streptokinase for survival after stroke.
- Accelerated tPA had fewer complications when compared to streptokinase, these included allergic reactions (1.6% vs. 5.8%), congestive heart failure (CHF) (15.2% vs. 16.8%), and atrioventricular (AV) block (7.3% vs. 8.7%).

STUDY CONCLUSIONS

Accelerated tPA combined with IV heparin was superior to the streptokinase regimens in reducing mortality and achieving net clinical benefit.

COMMENTARY

This study compared key initial approaches to acute MI at a time when few therapeutic options had demonstrated any effect on mortality. Current recommendations that universally favor the use of modern thrombolytics if rapid PCI is not available resulted from a serial of clinical trials that followed this study. Prior to this study, streptokinase was the main thrombolytic used in acute MI and subcutaneous heparin had been used with no added benefit. This study's large, factorial design provided robust evidence that combination therapy with heparin and thrombolytics reduces mortality and that accelerated thrombolytics provide an incremental benefit over the traditional streptokinase. Even though the risk of intracranial bleeding is not negligible for accelerated thrombolytics (1.5% incidence of stroke), the mortality benefits of therapy still favored treatment. This study showed that accelerated tPA, administered over a period of 1.5 hours, has the benefit of saving 10 additional lives per 1,000 and reduces the incidence of death and disabling stroke by 9 per 1,000 patients. The benefit of accelerated tPA also set the stage for the time-sensitive nature of thrombolysis that led to national recommendations for treatment within 30 minutes.

Question

Does the choice of agent used for fibrinolysis impact outcomes in patients with acute MI? Should heparin be coadministered with fibrinolytic agents?

Answer

Yes, for patients presenting within 6 hours of symptom onset, the coadministration of tPA and heparin leads to the largest reduction in mortality.

CHAPTER 24
PCI VS. LYTICS IN ACUTE MI: THE GUSTO IIB TRIAL

A Clinical Trial Comparing Primary Coronary Angioplasty With Tissue Plasminogen Activator for Acute Myocardial Infarction. The Global Use of Strategies to Open Occluded Coronary Arteries in Acute Coronary Syndromes (GUSTO IIb) Angioplasty Substudy Investigators

N Engl J Med. 1997;336(23):1621–1628

BACKGROUND
Coronary angioplasty was first developed in Switzerland in the late 1970s and rapidly spread. Before the late 1990s, tissue plasminogen activator (tPA) was the standard of care for patients who presented with acute MI. Prior to this study, it was widely known that prompt reperfusion improved clinical outcomes but there was little data concerning the effectiveness of tPA in comparison to angioplasty.

OBJECTIVES
To compare the effectiveness of primary percutaneous coronary intervention (PCI) or angioplasty to thrombolytics with antithrombotics (heparin and hirudin).

METHODS
Randomized controlled trial conducted in 57 hospitals experienced in angioplasty in nine countries in 1994 and 1995.

Participants
1,138 patients presenting within 12 hours of symptom onset and who had chest pain with 0.2-mV ST elevations in two or more leads or a left bundle. Select exclusion criteria: Taking warfarin, history of stroke, renal insufficiency, SBP >200 or DBP >110.

Intervention Evaluated
All patients were given standard medical therapy including aspirin and then were randomized to either angioplasty or accelerated tPA (bolus dosing followed by a 90-minute infusion) with either heparin or hirudin (as part of the larger GUSTO IIB trial).

Outcomes
Primary outcome was a composite outcome of death, nonfatal reinfarction and nonfatal disabling stroke.

KEY RESULTS
- There was a 9.6% incidence of the composite of death, reinfarction, or disabling stroke at 30 days in the angioplasty group as compared to 13.6% in the tPA group.

- There was no significant difference in death ($p = 0.37$), reinfarction ($p = 0.13$), or disabling stroke ($p = 0.11$) alone, though all demonstrated a trend toward improvement with angioplasty.
- Restoration of normal flow was obtained in 73% to 85% of angioplasty patients (depending on the group judging) with a steep drop in mortality (21.4% to 1.6%) if good flow was obtained.
- Angioplasty performed better in patients with <4 hours of time from the onset of symptoms to hospital arrival.

STUDY CONCLUSIONS

Patients treated with angioplasty had a mild but significant improvement in a composite end point of death, reinfarction, or disabling stroke when compared with patients treated with tPA.

COMMENTARY

This study was one of the major randomized controlled trials that established the benefit of PCI compared to thrombolysis in noncardiology research centers. It effectively established PCI as the standard of care for acute MI. Further, these results also provided early evidence for the "time is muscle" theory regarding the benefits of early reperfusion. This study's failure to find outcome benefits for PCI for specific end points may reflect the relatively primitive nature of interventional cardiology at the time: Only 5% of patients received stents at the time and long-term postintervention anticoagulation or antiplatelet therapy was not standard in this study.

Question

Is PCI superior to thrombolysis for patients with acute MI?

Answer

Yes, in comparison to thrombolysis, PCI reduces the 30-day composite outcome of death, reinfarction, or stroke.

CHAPTER 25: PCI TIMING IN ACS

Early Invasive vs. Selectively Invasive Management for Acute Coronary Syndromes
de Winter RJ, Windhausen F, Cornel JH, et al. *N Engl J Med.* 2005;353:1095–1104

BACKGROUND
Acute Coronary Syndromes (ACS) is a leading cause of mortality and morbidity in the United States and Percutaneous Coronary Intervention (PCI) has been a revolutionary advancement in the treatment of ACS. At the time of this study, guidelines recommend early PCI for patients with ACS without ST-segment elevation and troponinemia; however, clinical trials at the time only provided mixed support for this recommendation due to varied results, different definitions of myocardial infarction, inadequate study methods, and a failure to include other advancements in diagnostic testing and medical therapy such as low-molecular-weight heparins, dual antiplatelet therapy, and high-dose statins.

OBJECTIVES
To test the hypothesis that a general early invasive strategy is superior to a selectively invasive strategy for patients with ACS without ST-segment elevation and/or with an elevated troponin Unstable angina/Non-ST segment elevated myocardial infarction (UA/NSTEMI).

METHODS
Prospective, multicenter randomized control study at 42 Dutch hospitals between 2001 and 2003.

Patients
1,200 patients, aged 18 to 80, with acute onset of new or rest angina in the preceding 24 hours, an elevated cardiac troponin, and either ischemic changes on EKG or a documented history of coronary artery disease (prior myocardial infarction, stenosis on coronary angiography, or positive stress test). Select exclusion criteria: ST-segment elevation MI in past 48 hours, cardiogenic shock, or contraindication for antithrombotic or anticoagulant therapy.

Intervention Evaluated
Patients were randomly assigned to an early or selective invasive strategy. Patients randomized to early invasive approach underwent angiography 24 to 48 hours after admission and intervention with stenting or Coronary Artery Bypass Grafting (CABG). All patients received medical optimization to include aspirin, heparin (UFH or LMWH), clopidogrel, atorvastatin, and abciximab at PCI if performed. Patients randomized to selective approach were scheduled to undergo angiography and subsequent revascularization if they had refractory angina despite optimal medical therapy, hemodynamic instability, malignant arrhythmia, or positive predischarge stress test.

Outcomes
The primary end point was a composite of death (from all causes), recurrent myocardial infarction, or rehospitalization for angina within 1 year. Secondary outcomes included major bleeding not related to CABG and incidence of angina after index hospitalization.

KEY RESULTS
- The cumulative rate of the composite primary end point within 1 year was 22.7% in the early invasive group and 21.2% in the selectively invasive group
- One-year mortality was equal (2.5%) in both groups
- The risk of myocardial infarction at 1 year was significantly higher in the early invasive group (15.0% vs. 10.0%)
- The incidence of myocardial infarction related to PCI or CABG was also significantly higher in the early invasive group (11.3% vs. 5.4%)
- The percentage of patients free from anginal symptoms was similar between both groups (86% and 87%)
- There was an increase of major bleeding not related to CABG in the early invasive group (3.1% vs. 1.7%). P value not reported for this secondary outcome

STUDY CONCLUSIONS
Early invasive treatment of UA/NSTEMI is not superior to selective strategy given optimized medical therapy.

COMMENTARY
The current guidelines from the American College of Cardiology/American Heart Association (ACC/AHA) recommend early angiography followed by revascularization in high-risk patients with UA/NSTEMI. The ICTUS[1] trial showed that an early invasive strategy was nonsuperior to a selective strategy in preventing death, recurrent MI, and rehospitalization for angina. It is important to note that the patients in this study received optimal medical therapy with dual antiplatelet therapy, heparin, and high-dose statin in both groups. Some have pointed to the small sample size and overall lower incidence of mortality in both groups suggesting lower-risk ACS patients, as potential limitations which could account for the nonsuperior outcome. Although, the role of early vs. selective strategy is still evolving, this study made it clear that offering patients medical optimization therapy was of vital importance while trying to understand how to select patients for PCI remains an area of active inquiry.

Question
Does early PCI improve outcomes in patients with unstable angina or NSTEMI?

Answer
No, while an early invasive strategy in high-risk patients does not reduce mortality it remains a Class X recommendation by ACC/AHA clinical guidelines.

Reference
1. de Winter R, et al. Early Invasive versus Selectively Invasive Management for Acute Coronary Syndromes. *N Engl J Med.* 2005;353:1095–1104.

CHAPTER 26: DELAYING DEFIBRILLATION FOR CPR IN CARDIAC ARREST

Delaying Defibrillation to Give Basic Cardiopulmonary Resuscitation to Patients With Out-of-Hospital Ventricular Fibrillation: A Randomized Trial
Wik L, Hansen TB, Fylling F, et al. *JAMA*. 2003;289(11):1389–1395

BACKGROUND
Immediate defibrillation was considered standard treatment for patients with out-of-hospital cardiac arrest (OHCA) secondary to ventricular fibrillation (VF). Two small studies, one dog model and one nonrandomized human trial, had suggested that prolonged VF was more responsive to defibrillation if CPR and epinephrine had been administered prior. Understanding this, there was a need to assess the benefit of early defibrillation with a randomized clinical trial in human subjects.

OBJECTIVES
To determine the efficacy of CPR before defibrillation in patients with VF.

METHODS
Nonblinded, randomized trial in an Emergency Medical Services (EMS) system of Norway.

Patients
Two hundred patients, age >18, with out-of-hospital VF or pulseless ventricular tachycardia (VT) in whom the ambulance personnel had not witnessed the cardiac arrest.

Intervention Evaluated
Patients were randomized after defibrillator electrocardiogram verification of VF/VT to receive either standard care with immediate defibrillation or 3 minutes of basic CPR by ambulance personnel prior to defibrillation. If initial defibrillation was unsuccessful, the standard group received 1 minute of CPR before additional defibrillation attempts compared with 3 minutes in the CPR first group.

Outcomes
Primary outcome was survival to hospital discharge. Secondary outcomes were hospital admission with return of spontaneous circulation (ROSC), 1-year survival, and neurologic outcome. A prespecified analysis examined subgroups with response times either lesser or greater than 5 minutes.

KEY RESULTS
- There were no differences in survival to hospital discharge, ROSC, or 1-year survival between each group.
- There was no difference in outcome between the two groups if the EMS response time was less than 5 minutes.

- With response times longer than 5 minutes:
  - More patients in the CPR first group achieved ROSC (**58%** [37/64] vs. **38%** [21/55])
  - More patients in the CPR first group survived to hospital discharge (**22%** [14/64] vs. **4%** [2/55])
  - Patients in the CPR first group had greater 1-year survival (**20%** [13/64] vs. **4%** [2/55])

STUDY CONCLUSIONS

Compared to immediate defibrillation, CPR prior to defibrillation offered no survival advantage for patients with OHCA due to VT/VF. However, the patients with response times longer than 5 minutes may have better outcomes with CPR prior to defibrillation.

COMMENTARY

While early defibrillation is a critical aspect of resuscitation efforts in patients with VF this large randomized study provided the first human subject results not subject to selection bias that showed a CPR first strategy may benefit a cohort of patients with prolonged VF. This trial challenged the standard of cardiac arrest care, suggesting that delayed defibrillation may improve outcomes; however, also highlighting the continued importance of early time to resuscitation including both defibrillation and high-quality CPR. This study was limited by its nonblinded design, which could have risked unequal resuscitation efforts between groups. The positive findings found for the secondary outcome also suggest that more work is required to determine the optimum time after which CPR first should be implemented, and how long CPR should be used before defibrillation in these cases. In summary, this paper helped show that resuscitation is more than a single act, such as CPR or defibrillation, but relies on timing and access to high-quality prehospital systems.

Question

Should CPR be performed prior to defibrillation in patients with VT/VF arrest?

Answer

Not necessarily, while CPR prior to defibrillation in the prehospital setting does not improve survival to hospital discharge, patients with delayed EMS response may benefit from receiving CPR first.

CHAPTER 27
THERAPEUTIC HYPOTHERMIA IN CARDIAC ARREST

Mild Therapeutic Hypothermia to Improve the Neurologic Outcome After Cardiac Arrest
Hypothermia After Cardiac Arrest Study Group. *N Engl J Med.* 2002;346(8):549–556

BACKGROUND
Cardiac arrest resulting in cerebral hypoperfusion frequently leads to severe neurologic morbidity and mortality. At the time of this study, only animal models and case report data showed compelling evidence of the benefit of therapeutic hypothermia following cardiac arrest. This study investigated whether mild hypothermia could lead to favorable neurologic outcomes in human subject resuscitation from out-of-hospital cardiac arrest.

OBJECTIVES
To determine the effect of mild hypothermia on neurologic outcome after cardiac arrest.

METHODS
Multicenter, randomized controlled trial at nine centers in five European countries between 1996 and 2001.

Patients
Two hundred and seventy five patients 18 to 75 years old. Inclusion criteria: Return of spontaneous circulation (ROSC) after witnessed cardiac arrest from ventricular fibrillation or nonperfusing ventricular tachycardia, estimated 5- to 15-minute interval from arrest to attempted resuscitation, and <60 minutes from collapse to ROSC. Select exclusion criteria: Temperature <30°C on admission, comatose state prior to arrest, pregnancy, response to verbal commands after ROSC and before randomization, persistent hypotension, or hypoxemia.

Intervention Evaluated
Therapeutic hypothermia (32°C to 34°C by bladder measurement) over 24 hours.

Outcomes
Primary outcomes were favorable neurologic outcome within 6 months and good recovery, or moderate disability defined as able to live independently and work at least part-time. Secondary outcomes included overall mortality at 6 months and the rate of complications during the first 7 days after cardiac arrest.

KEY RESULTS
- Fifty five percent (75/136) hypothermic patients had a favorable outcome compared to 40% (54/137) of normothermic patients; a risk ratio of 1.4.
- Six-month mortality in hypothermic group was 41% compared to 55% in normothermic group.
- There was no significant difference in complication rate between the groups.

STUDY CONCLUSIONS

Patients successfully resuscitated after cardiac arrest and treated with mild hypothermia had more favorable neurologic outcome and reduced 6-month mortality when compared to normothermic patients.

COMMENTARY

This large trial provided strong evidence that therapeutic hypothermia improves mortality and neurologic outcomes. In addition to clinical outcomes, the authors posit that the impact of mild therapeutic hypothermia in public health terms is also significant. Using the estimate of 375,000 cardiac arrests per year in Europe, this study suggests that therapeutic hypothermia would improve neurologic outcome in 1,200 to 7,500 patients resulting in improved quality of life and both direct and indirect cost savings. Limitations of the study include narrow inclusion criteria (only 8% of the patients screened looks good were eligible for the trial), and treatment physicians were not blinded, which may have added to more vigilance with regard to all resuscitation efforts in the intervention group. Since this study, mild therapeutic hypothermia has become standard of care in the postresuscitative period for cardiac arrest patients, but research continues into appropriate timing and temperature targets.[1,2]

Question

Does therapeutic hypothermia improve outcomes in cardiac arrest patients?

Answer

Yes, mild therapeutic hypothermia for select patients results in improved neurologic outcomes and decreased mortality at 6 months.[3]

References

1. Kim F, et al. Effect of prehospital induction of mild hypothermia on survival and neurological status among adults with cardiac arrest: a randomized clinical trial. *JAMA*. 2014;311(1):45–52.
2. Nielsen N, et al. Targeted temperature management at 33°C versus 36°C after cardiac arrest. *N Engl J Med*. 2013;369(23):2197–2206.
3. Hazinski MF, Field JM. "2010 American Heart Association Guidelines for Cardiopulmonary Resuscitation and Emergency Cardiovascular Care Science." *Circulation*. 2010;122(Suppl):S639–S946.

CHAPTER 28
CPR QUALITY IN OUT-OF-HOSPITAL CARDIAC ARREST

Quality of Cardiopulmonary Resuscitation During Out-of-Hospital Cardiac Arrest
Wik L, Kramer-Johansen J, Myklebust H, et al. *JAMA*. 2005;293(3):299–304

BACKGROUND
Since standards and guidelines were first published almost 38 years ago for cardiopulmonary resuscitation (CPR), countless health care professionals have been trained in CPR. Studies have shown that outcomes in cardiac arrest improve with higher-quality CPR.[1] Unfortunately, other studies show that a knowledge gap exists regarding quality of CPR in real-life cardiac arrest scenarios despite training.[2]

OBJECTIVES
To measure the quality of out-of-hospital CPR performed by ambulance personnel, as measured by adherence to CPR guidelines.

METHODS
Case series looking at cardiac arrests in three European regions.

Participants
One hundred and seventy-six patients, >18 years old, with out-of-hospital cardiac arrest between March 2002 and October 2003.

Intervention
Standard defibrillators were fitted with a second chest pad that had an accelerometer and a pressure sensor. These modified defibrillators were placed on six ambulances and recorded the quality of chest compressions and ventilations.

Outcomes
Adherence to international guidelines for CPR. Target values were 100 to 120 compressions per minute with a depth of 1.5 to 2 in and two ventilations for every 15 compressions before intubation.

KEY RESULTS
- Chest compressions were not delivered 48% of the time that the patient was in cardiac arrest. When the time for EKG analysis and defibrillation was subtracted the percentage of time without chest compressions was 38%.
- The mean compression rate was 64/min.
- Only 28% of the compressions reached the goal depth of 1.5 to 2 in.
- A mean of 11 breaths were given per minute.
- Thirty-five percent of patients (61) had return of spontaneous circulation and five out of six patients discharged alive from hospital had normal neurologic outcomes.

STUDY CONCLUSIONS
Chest compressions were not delivered half of the time in out-of-hospital CPR and most were too shallow, demonstrating opportunity to improve the quality of out-of-hospital CPR.

> ### COMMENTARY
> High-quality CPR has long been the cornerstone of out-of-hospital strategies to improve survival from cardiac arrest. Furthermore, the successful use of increasingly available out-of-hospital defibrillation technology also requires high-quality CPR. In real-life scenarios, as this study proves, there often are long periods without any chest compressions and shallow compression depth. These findings are observational and cannot be interpreted to directly improve outcomes; however, they demonstrate the real-world challenges of delivering effective CPR. This study focused attention on the need for improved out-of-hospital CPR and laid the groundwork for the changes reflected in the 2010 American Heart Association (AHA) guidelines which went from A-B-C (Airway, Breathing, Compressions) to C-A-B (Compressions, Airway, Breathing).

Question
How effective is out-of-hospital CPR for patients arriving to the ED in cardiac arrest?

Answer
Many patients do not receive CPR while in cardiac arrest, and of those that do, many receive inadequate CPR. High-quality CPR is 100 compressions per minute and a depth of 2 in per compression.

References
1. Van Hoeyweghen RJ, Bossaert LL, Mullie A, et al. Belgian Cerebral Resuscitation Study Group. Quality and efficiency of bystander CPR. *Resuscitation*. 1993;26:47–52.
2. Donnelly P, Assar D, Lester C. A comparison of manikin CPR performance by lay persons trained in three variations of basic life support guidelines. *Resuscitation*. 2000;45:195–199.

CHAPTER 29
CHEST COMPRESSION ONLY CPR

Cardiopulmonary Resuscitation by Chest Compression Alone or With Mouth-to-Mouth Ventilation
Hallstrom A, Cobb L, Johnson E, et al. *N Engl J Med.* 2000;342(21):1546–1553

BACKGROUND
Prior to this study, it was a dogma that CPR provided by all persons included both chest compressions and interruptions for rescue breaths. Bystander-initiated CPR showed a mortality improvement of around 50% but was limited in cases where bystanders did not know how to do CPR. A prior study had demonstrated the value of dispatcher-instructed CPR but it took an average of 2.4 minutes to deliver the instructions. The most common reason CPR was not initiated was that Emergency Medical Services (EMS) had already arrived by completion of the instructions.

OBJECTIVES
To determine if changing the dispatcher instructions to have bystanders perform chest compressions without interruptions for ventilation would yield at least a 3.5% absolute increase in survival to hospital discharge.

METHODS
Prospective randomized controlled trial conducted in a single metropolitan US city EMS system.

Participants
Five hundred and twenty patients who were unconscious or not breathing normally for whom 911 was called. Select exclusion criteria: CPR already in progress or planned, known drug or alcohol intoxication, or traumatic arrest.

Intervention Evaluated
Dispatcher-instructed bystander CPR with chest compressions only.

Outcomes
The primary outcome was survival to hospital discharge. Secondary outcomes were survival to hospital admission and neurologic status at hospital discharge (no morbidity, impaired but able to perform daily activities independently, requiring some assistance with daily activities, or completely dependent).

KEY RESULTS
- Time to EMS arrival (4 minutes) and initial rhythm (approximately 40% ventricular fibrillation) were similar in both groups.

- CPR instructions were completely delivered in 81% ($n = 83$) of the treatment group vs. 62% ($n = 68$) of the control group.
- The treatment group had a higher rate of survival to admission (40.2% vs. 34.1%) and discharge (14.6% vs. 10.4%), although neither outcome was statistically significant (p-values 0.15 and 0.18, respectively).
- There were no significant differences in neurologic status.

STUDY CONCLUSIONS

A strategy of dispatcher-instructed chest compressions plus ventilations did not perform better than chest compressions alone. Patients receiving chest compressions only had a trend toward higher rates of survival to admission and discharge, although statistical significance was not reached.

COMMENTARY

This study demonstrated that bystanders instructed by dispatchers successfully followed instructions for chest compression-only CPR a greater percentage of the time and patients did not have demonstrably worse survival or outcomes. Study strengths include effective randomization and rigorous methodology regarding the details of the instruction provided by the dispatcher. However, statistical significance was not reached and despite the stated conclusion, this study was not designed a priori to be a noninferiority trial. Large numbers of patients were excluded due to conditions such as stroke, seizure, and syncope being initially misclassified as cardiac arrest, so an intention-to-treat analysis was not performed. This study was also performed in a highly efficient EMS system with average response times of 4 minutes and the conclusions may not be generalizable to systems with longer delays in arrival. The authors did demonstrate that their intervention was safe and was performed successfully a greater percentage of the time than the current standard of care (p-value was not reported). This study showed the potential effect of changes in prehospital CPR on outcomes and paved the way for prioritizing circulation above breathing, as espoused in current "C-B-A" guidelines.

Question
How can bystander CPR improve patient survival from cardiac arrest?

Answer
Dispatcher-instructed chest compression-only CPR improved bystander CPR rates without increasing adverse events in the absence of ventilation.

CHAPTER 30

AMIODARONE IN VENTRICULAR FIBRILLATION

Amiodarone as Compared with Lidocaine for Shock-resistant Ventricular Fibrillation
Dorian P, Cass D, Schwartz B, et al. *N Engl J Med.* 2002;346:884–890

BACKGROUND
Ventricular fibrillation (VF) is a commonly encountered rhythm and often the most survivable form of out-of-hospital cardiac arrests. Some cases are resistant to conversion by defibrillation, and the addition of pharmacologic antiarrhythmics to defibrillation has become the standard of care supported by clinical guidelines for refractory VF. At the time of this study, lidocaine was the drug of choice for refractory VF; however, little evidence supported its use. This study compares amiodarone to lidocaine for shock-resistant VF.

OBJECTIVES
To compare the efficacy and mortality associated with the use of amiodarone when compared to lidocaine in shock-resistant VF in out-of-hospital cardiac arrests.

METHODS
Double-blinded, randomized trial done in the Toronto Emergency Medical Services (EMS) system between 1991 and 2001.

Participants
Three hundred and forty-seven patients with a mean age of 67. Inclusion criteria: Documented out-of-hospital VF not due to trauma or with other cardiac rhythms that converted to VF or if VF was resistant to three shocks from an external defibrillator or if VF was recurrent after successful initial defibrillation.

Intervention
Paramedics were given kits with either amiodarone or lidocaine in randomized order.

Outcomes
The primary endpoint was survival to hospital admission. Patients who died in the ED were not considered to have been admitted. Secondary outcomes included survival to discharge and adverse events such as need to administer atropine or dopamine after drug delivery.

KEY RESULTS
- Mean interval from the time at which paramedics were dispatched to the time of their arrival was 7 ± 3 minutes. Mean time to drug administration was 25 ± 8 minutes.

- After treatment with amiodarone, 22.8% of 180 patients survived to hospital admission as compared with 12% of the 167 patients treated with lidocaine.
- Amongst patients for whom the time from dispatch to drug administration was equal or less than the median (24 minutes), 27.7% of those given amiodarone compared to 15.3% of those given lidocaine survived to hospital admission ($p = 0.05$).
- After adjustment for other factors, the only factors that significantly influenced the primary outcome were the study drug assignment, the length of time to administration of drug, and the presence or absence of a transient return of spontaneous circulation (ROSC).

CONCLUSIONS

In out-of-hospital shock-resistant VF, amiodarone when compared to lidocaine led to a greater number of patients surviving to hospital admission.

COMMENTARY

While clinical guidelines supported the use of drugs in addition to shocks there had been no comparative clinical trials for the most common and most survivable rhythm—VF. This study shows clear superiority of amiodarone over lidocaine in shock-resistant VF. In fact, this was the first randomized study to show the benefit of any drug over placebo in patients with out-of-hospital cardiac arrest. Patients who received the drug quicker and had intermittent ROSC also did better. The study was also unique as it used an active comparator and blinding/concealment with paramedics which was likely to be very effective. However, this study was conducted in a Toronto EMS system with rapid response times and the study outcome, survival to hospital admission (not discharge or long term), may not be clinically meaningful to many patients. The study was conducted from 1998 to 2001 and is relevant as the current and revised 2010 ACLS guidelines emphasize the CAB algorithm as opposed to the ABC algorithm with definite airway management getting a secondary priority to aggressive management of shockable rhythms. Thus, with the current guidelines, amiodarone would have been delivered quicker, and potentially impart more of a survival benefit and theoretically increase survival to hospital discharge.

Question
Is there a survival advantage to using amiodarone instead of lidocaine in shock-resistant ventricular fibrillation?

Answer
Yes, in comparison to lidocaine, amiodarone increases survival to hospital admission.

CHAPTER 31: EPINEPHRINE IN CARDIAC ARREST

A Comparison of Repeated High Doses and Repeated Standard Doses of Epinephrine for Cardiac Arrest Outside the Hospital
Gueugniaud PY, Mols P, Goldstein P, et al. *N Engl J Med.* 1998;339(22):1595–1601

BACKGROUND
Epinephrine has long been the first-choice agent for blood pressure support in patients with cardiac arrest. Prior to this study there had been significant evidence that higher doses of epinephrine improved myocardial and cerebral blood flow. Small studies had never confirmed a significant effect on patient mortality in cardiac arrest.

OBJECTIVES
To compare the efficacy of low-dose (1 mg repeated) vs. high-dose (5 mg) epinephrine in adults with out-of-hospital cardiac arrest.

METHODS
Randomized, controlled trial conducted in 12 European centers between 1994 and 1996.

Participants
1,667 patients found to be ventricular fibrillation refractory to shocks, pulseless electrical activity, or asystole. Select exclusion criteria: Patients with traumatic arrest, obvious signs of irreversible death, or prior epinephrine administration.

Intervention
During resuscitation, the treatment group received up to 15 doses of 5 mg of epinephrine whereas patients in the control group received up to 15 doses of 1 mg of epinephrine all at 3-minute intervals. Providers were blinded.

Outcomes
The primary endpoints were return of spontaneous circulation (ROSC), survival to hospital admission, and survival to hospital discharge. Secondary endpoints included neurologic function on discharge from the hospital assessed using the Glasgow Coma Scale early and then a cerebral performance scale at hospital discharge (ranging from normal-to-slight disability to brain dead).

KEY RESULTS
- There was a small but significant decrease in ROSC in the high-dose epinephrine group compared with the standard arm (38% vs. 34.3%).
- There was a smaller difference in survival to hospital admission in the high-dose epinephrine group compared to the standard arm (25.3% vs. 22.7%, $p = 0.05$).

- There was no significant difference in 24-hour survival, survival to hospital discharge, or neurologic outcome at the time of discharge between the two groups.
- Patients who had witnessed arrests had improved ROSC (45.2% vs. 40.1%) and survival to ICU admission (29.2% vs. 26.1%) in the high-dose group compared with the standard-dose group.

STUDY CONCLUSIONS

High-dose epinephrine given in repeated doses during the treatment of out-of-hospital arrest resulted in a significant improvement in ROSC and survival to hospital arrival; however, there was no significant benefit on survival to hospital discharge or neurologic outcomes.

COMMENTARY

Long-term survival and recovery of neurologic function in patients who have out-of-hospital cardiac arrest is rare and is even worse for patients who present with nonshockable rhythms. This study examined a modification to standard therapy that showed some promise of improved outcomes. Uniquely, this study was able to do this in a random, blinded fashion. While high-dose epinephrine does provide some benefits in the short term as measured by ROSC and survival to presentation to the hospital, there appears to be little benefit in terms of more patient-oriented outcomes such as survival to hospital discharge or neurologic outcome. This study reinforces the current ACLS dosing of epinephrine of 1 mg every 3 to 5 minutes for patients with sudden cardiac arrest.

Question

Does high-dose epinephrine improve outcomes in cardiac arrest patients?

Answer

Minimally, high-dose epinephrine increases the likelihood of return of spontaneous circulation and survival to hospital admission, but does not improve survival to hospital discharge.

CHAPTER 32 tPA IN PEA CARDIAC ARREST

Tissue Plasminogen Activator in Cardiac Arrest with Pulseless Electrical Activity
Abu-Laban RB, Christenson JM, Innes GD, et al. *N Engl J Med.* 2002;346(20):
1522–1528

BACKGROUND
Out-of-hospital cardiac arrest accounts for 250,000 deaths annually with pulseless electrical activity (PEA) the presenting rhythm in 20% of arrests. The survival rate to discharge in these cases is 4%. Coronary and pulmonary thromboembolism frequently present with PEA as the initial rhythm. It was postulated that because fibrinolytics show marked benefits in both acute MI and PE they may improve the low survival rates in PEA arrest. Several case series and nonrandomized trials had lent support to this idea, and this study was designed to more rigorously assess these claims.

OBJECTIVES
To evaluate the effect of tPA during CPR in adults with undifferentiated PEA (i.e., with an unknown or presumed cardiovascular cause) that was not responsive to initial therapy.

METHODS
Double-blinded, randomized placebo-controlled trial conducted in Canada at seven advanced life support paramedic base stations and three tertiary teaching hospital emergency departments between February 1998 and September 1999.

Participants
Two hundred and thirty-three patients age >16 with PEA for more than 1 minute and no palpable pulse for more than 3 minutes. Select exclusion criteria: Trauma, overdose, pregnancy, history of intracranial tumor or hemorrhage, evidence of tension pneumothorax or cardiac tamponade or if a paramedic student was directing resuscitation.

Intervention
Patients were randomly assigned to receive treatment either with placebo or tPA. Both were infused over 15 minutes and the resuscitation continued for another 15 minutes.

Outcomes
Primary outcome was survival to hospital discharge. Secondary outcomes were return of spontaneous circulation, length of hospital stay, hemorrhage, and neurologic outcome.

KEY RESULTS
- One patient in the tPA group survived to hospital discharge as compared with none in the placebo group.
- There was no difference in the proportion of patients with ROSC (21.4% in the tPA group and 23.3% in the placebo group).

CONCLUSIONS
In patients with undifferentiated PEA arrest, the administration of tPA did not offer a survival benefit over placebo.

COMMENTARY
Despite the high mortality of PEA-associated cardiac arrests, there are no universal medical treatments for this entity. This study was able to study this rare disease in a randomized, controlled fashion with a fairly large sample size in the prehospital setting. However, out of 756 patients with a qualifying episode of PEA, only 233 were eligible and over 50% of these had an initial rhythm of ventricular fibrillation or asystole. Only 48.7% of patients in the tPA group had an initial rhythm of PEA as compared to 57.8% in the placebo group. As a result, the study may have been underpowered to detect a clinical effect in patients with predominantly PEA arrest. In addition, the study was conducted between 1998 and 1999 with significant proportions of the tPA group getting therapies such as sodium bicarbonate, lidocaine, atropine–all of which are no longer a part of standard ACLS protocols for PEA today. While this study broadly concluded that tPA is not beneficial for patients with out-of-hospital PEA arrest due possibly to a low prevalence of thromboembolic etiology, more recent work is beginning to suggest a benefit for selective tPA in patients with a higher probability of cardiopulmonary-driven PEA arrest.

Question
Does the empiric use of tPA improve outcomes in patients with PEA arrest?

Answer
No, in undifferentiated PEA arrest patients the use of fibrinolysis did not improve survival.

CHAPTER 33
VASOPRESSIN VS. EPINEPHRINE FOR CARDIAC ARREST

Vasopressin vs. Epinephrine for Inhospital Cardiac Arrest: A Randomized Controlled Trial
Steill IG, Hébert PC, Wells GA, et al. *Lancet.* 2001;358(9276):105–109

BACKGROUND
With an estimated 300,000 cardiac arrests in North America annually, and only a 6% survival among those requiring epinephrine, there is great room to improve survival. A small study preceding this work showed a significant survival benefit in out-of-hospital cardiac arrest patients treated with vasopressin vs. epinephrine. This study looked to formally evaluate vasopressin as an alternative to epinephrine in a randomized controlled design in the inpatient setting.

OBJECTIVES
To compare the efficacy of vasopressin to epinephrine in the inpatient cardiac arrest setting.

METHODS
Triple-blinded, randomized trial in the EDs, critical care units and wards of three Canadian teaching hospitals.

Participants
Two hundred patients, >16 years old, who were admitted to hospital, had a cardiac arrest, and required epinephrine according to the AHA ACLS protocols for asystole, PEA, or refractory VF. Select exclusion criteria: Prehospital cardiac arrest, exsanguination, and trauma. One hundred and four patients were assigned to the vasopressin arm and 96 to epinephrine.

Intervention
Patients received one dose of vasopressin or epinephrine intravenously as the initial vasopressor during ACLS. Patients who failed to respond to the study intervention were given epinephrine as a rescue medication.

Outcomes
Primary outcomes were survival to hospital discharge, survival to 1 hour, and neurologic function. Preplanned subgroup assessments of patients with MI or infarction, initial cardiac rhythm, and age were also done.

KEY RESULTS
For patients receiving vasopressin or epinephrine
- There was no statistically significant difference between the vasopressin and epinephrine group in survival to hospital discharge (12% vs. 14%, $p = 0.67$) or 1-hour survival (39% vs. 35%, $p = 0.66$).
- Survivors also had similar median mini-mental state examination scores–36 (range = 19 to 38) in the vasopressin vs. 35 (20 to 40) in the epinephrine group, $p = 0.75$ and median cerebral performance category scores (1 vs. 1).

CONCLUSIONS
For inpatient cardiac arrest patients, there is no survival advantage of using vasopressin over epinephrine as the initial vasopressor.

COMMENTARY
Vasopressin has been studied as an adjunctive or monotherapy alternative to various adrenergic agonists in critical illness. This study was the first evaluate vasopressin in comparison with epinephrine which is the longest standing vasoactive treatment in cardiac arrest. This study was well designed and included a variety of elements to ensure the random allocation of treatment assignment as well as blinding of the treating providers and in outcome ascertainment. The study was also appropriately powered with an adequate sample size to be the definitive work demonstrating no benefit in either survival or neurologic outcomes with the use of vasopressin rather than epinephrine for hospital patients with cardiac arrest. In a larger sense of cardiac arrest care and resuscitation, the study also highlights that survival is poor in cardiac arrest and that it would seem implausible that a single drug alone could impact major outcomes such as neurologic function. It does not appear from these results that vasopressin is significantly worse than epinephrine for patients with undifferentiated cardiac arrest. As such this study's findings are reflected in the AHA guidelines and ACLS recommendations to use vasopressin as an alternative therapy for inpatient cardiac arrest patients.

Question
Is there a benefit to vasopressin over epinephrine in the inpatient who suffers a cardiac arrest?

Answer
No, for undifferentiated inpatient cardiac arrest, there is no survival benefit or improvement in neurologic outcomes with the use of vasopressin over epinephrine.

CHAPTER 34: PILL-IN-THE-POCKET APPROACH FOR ATRIAL FIBRILLATION

Outpatient Treatment of Recent-onset Atrial Fibrillation with the "Pill-in-the-Pocket" Approach
Alboni P, Botto GL, Baldi N, et al. *N Engl J Med.* 2004;351(23):2384–2391

BACKGROUND
Recurrent episodes of paroxysmal atrial fibrillation are responsible for a large number of ED visits, many of them by otherwise healthy people who only have a few events each year. Radiofrequency ablation is only used in patients who have frequent arrhythmic episodes despite long-term oral prophylaxis. This excludes a category of patients with infrequent and typically well-tolerated episodes. Pharmacologic cardioversion mechanisms such as propafenone and flecainide have proven safe, effective, and timely in converting atrial fibrillation in the inpatient settings. However, no studies examined patient directed, at home therapy as an alternative to hospital admission.

OBJECTIVES
This study attempted to determine if a single dose of patient-administered antiarrhythmic such as propafenone or flecainide could be used to cardiovert a limited subset of patients to sinus rhythm in the outpatient setting.

METHODS
Prospective comparative therapeutic study in Italy between 2001 and 2003.

Participants
Two hundred and ten patients, of the 268 screened, treated their atrial fibrillation at home. Inclusion criteria: 18 to 75 year olds who presented to the ED with EKG-confirmed atrial fibrillation, a heart rate greater than 70, and a systolic blood pressure greater than 100. Select exclusion criteria: Structural heart disease, prior long episodes (>7 days) of fibrillation, ischemia, cardiomyopathy, heart failure, previous second- or third-degree AV block, or prophylactic antiarrhythmic treatment at presentation.

Intervention Evaluated
Subjects were cardioverted with the clinician's choice of a standard dose of propafenone or flecainide and then monitored as an inpatient. If successfully converted to sinus rhythm, patients then received outpatient treatment with the same, taking it after 5 minutes of symptoms. They were told to call the ED if their symptoms did not resolve within 6 hours or came back within 24 hours.

Outcomes
The primary endpoint was successful treatment and the rate of adverse events. The secondary outcome was the number of ED visits or hospital admissions for these patients.

KEY RESULTS
- About 12% of all patients who presented in atrial fibrillation were found to be candidates for this study; they had an average of three episodes per year.
- Both propafenone and flecainide were found to be 94% effective in the outpatient setting for converting atrial fibrillation.
- There were 59.8 events/month in the group for the year prior to enrollment compared with 54.5 events/month for the year after. Though there were 618 episodes of atrial fibrillation during the study period, only 26 (5%) episodes required a trip to the ED for further intervention.
- Thirteen percent of patients had to leave the study due to: Drug ineffectiveness (6%), multiple recurrent episodes of fibrillation (3%), noncompliance (5%), or side effects including RVR (2%).

STUDY CONCLUSIONS
Outpatient administration of propafenone or flecainide to treat atrial fibrillation is safe and effective, with 94% of patients pharmacologically cardioverted successfully every time they went into fibrillation. An outpatient treatment strategy greatly reduces the ED utilization of these patients.

COMMENTARY
Many ED visits for symptomatic atrial fibrillation result in electrical cardioversion without any further intervention. This study showed that immediate chemical cardioversion is a safe and effective method for healthy patients. Chemical cardioversion is often cheaper, does not expose the patient to the risks of procedural sedation and requires less provider time. In addition, subsequent outpatient use of these antiarrhythmics sharply reduced ED visits for these patients. However, it is important to remember that only a very small proportion of those examined met the inclusion criteria so the practical applications may be limited.

Question
Is it safe to discharge patients with paroxysmal atrial fibrillation with an oral antiarrhythmic to treat future episodes outside of the ED or clinic?

Answer
Yes, patients can be safely treated for *symptomatic* atrial fibrillation with a single-dose oral arrhythmic if they are carefully selected and the treatment has been proven to benefit them.

CHAPTER 35
RHYTHM CONTROL IN ATRIAL FIBRILLATION: THE AFFIRM TRIAL

A Comparison of Rate Control and Rhythm Control in Patients with Atrial Fibrillation
Wyse DG, Waldo AL, DiMarco JP, et al. *N Engl J Med.* 2002;347:1825–1833

BACKGROUND
The management of atrial fibrillation has centered around two main strategies–rate control that allowed atrial fibrillation to persist or rhythm control with prompt return to normal sinus rhythm via cardioversion or the use of antiarrhythmic drugs. Until this study, no large scale comparative trials of these two strategies existed.

OBJECTIVES
To compare the long-term effects of rate vs. rhythm control for patients with atrial fibrillation.

METHODS
Randomized, controlled trial conducted across 213 clinic sites within the University of Washington.

Participants
4,060 patients, >65 years old, with atrial fibrillation likely to be recurrent and likely to cause illness or death. Inclusion criteria: Long treatment for atrial fibrillation was indicated, anticoagulation was not contraindicated, the patient was eligible to undergo trials of at least two drugs in both treatment strategies.

Intervention
In the rhythm-control strategy–the treating physician chose an antiarrhythmic drug from a variety of options. Attempts to maintain sinus rhythm could include cardioversion as necessary. In the rate-control strategy–beta blockers, calcium channel blockers, digoxin, and/or combination of these drugs were used to control heart rate. The goal resting heart rate was 80 and goal activity heart rate at the end of a 6-minute walk was 110 beats per minute.

Outcomes
The primary endpoint was overall mortality. A composite secondary endpoint comprised death, disabling stroke, disabling anoxic encephalopathy, major bleeding, and cardiac arrest.

KEY RESULTS
- Three hundred and fifty-six deaths among the patients assigned to rhythm control and 310 deaths among those assigned to rate control.

- Mortality at 5 years was 23.8% in the rhythm-control group and 21.3% in the rate-control group; hazard ratio, was 1.15; $p = 0.08$.
- More patients in the rhythm-control group were hospitalized (1,374–rhythm vs. 1,220–rate) and had adverse drug reactions prompting discontinuation of the drug–414 (rhythm) vs. 176 (rate).
- The majority of strokes that occurred were after warfarin had been stopped or when the International Normalized Ratio (INR) was subtherapeutic.

CONCLUSIONS

Rhythm control in this specific and rather sick patient cohort offers no survival advantage over rate control and is associated with higher adverse drug reactions. Anticoagulation should be continued in both groups of patients.

COMMENTARY

This study is unique since this is a large comparative, noninferiority trial with good long-term outcomes. This trial showed that patients did not need cardioversion and that rate control combined with strict anticoagulation therapy was preferred in the populations studied. This meant that emergency physicians did not need to make rhythm conversion a priority and thereby reduced the need for unnecessary cardioversions, which carry unique risks. The study is confounded by the significant degree of crossover in both directions with subjects going from rhythm control to rate control and vice versa. In addition, exploratory subgroup findings show great variance in hazard ratios based on different variables such as initial rhythm, age, comorbidities etc., which may suggest that rhythm control would be optimal for select populations. Ultimately, this study resulted in general shift away from the use of antiarrhythmic for atrial fibrillation, which changed both the types of presentations evaluated and the subsequent disposition of ED patients.

Question

Is there a survival advantage to rhythm control vs. rate control in patients with atrial fibrillation?

Answer

No, the majority of patients with recurrent atrial fibrillation can be safely managed with adequate rate control and anticoagulation therapy.

CHAPTER 36 RISK OF STROKE IN ATRIAL FIBRILLATION CARDIOVERSION

Risk for Clinical Thromboembolism Associated with Conversion to Sinus Rhythm in Patients with Atrial Fibrillation Lasting Less Than 48 Hours
Weigner MJ, Caulfield TA, Danias PG, et al. *Ann Intern Med.* 1997;126(8):615–620

BACKGROUND
Atrial fibrillation (AFib) is the most common arrhythmia and a common reason for presentation to the ED. Rhythm control with cardioversion is recommended but carries an estimated 5% to 7% risk of thromboembolism. Before this study, the risk of thromboembolism in a patient who presented less than 48 hours after onset was assumed to be low; however, some studies had suggested that up to 14% of patients with AFib <3 days developed cardiac thrombus.

OBJECTIVES
To determine the incidence of cardioversion-related thromboembolism in patients presenting with onset of AFib less than 48 hours.

METHODS
Prospective, observational cohort conducted at two US academic medical centers from 1990 to 1996.

Patients
Three hundred and seventy-five of 1,822 screened patients were included based on onset of AFib less than 48 hours prior to presentation. Select exclusion criteria: Indeterminate onset of AFib, evidence of thromboembolism on initial presentation, or current therapeutic anticoagulation.

Intervention Evaluated
Active chemical and/or electrical cardioversion to normal sinus rhythm.

Outcomes
Primary outcome was clinical thromboembolic event including cerebrovascular accident (CVA), transient ischemic attack (TIA), and peripheral arterial embolism following cardioversion.

KEY RESULTS
- 95.2% (357 patients) converted to sinus rhythm and 0.8% (three patients) had a thromboembolic event.
- Majority (66.7%) of patients converted spontaneously; no report of modality used in other 28.5% of patients that were actively converted.

STUDY CONCLUSIONS

The incidence of thromboembolism in patients presenting within 48 hours of onset of AFib is low, which makes early cardioversion a safe therapy to consider in the management of these patients.

> **COMMENTARY**
>
> The aim of this study was to estimate the risk of thromboembolism in the treatment of AFib with cardioversion in patients presenting within 48 hours of onset. Prior to this study clinicians had no estimate of real risk in this patient population leading to admission for prolonged anticoagulation and/or transesophageal echocardiogram to detect atrial thrombus prior to attempted cardioversion. This study is unique in its prospective design and showed conclusively that early cardioversion of uncomplicated AFib of less than 48 hours duration is safe. This study[1] helped inform the consensus statements by the AHA/ACC informing clinical guidelines on the management of AFib. More recently, the Ottawa Aggressive Protocol,[2] suggests that low-risk patients in the ED can be safely converted with IV procainamide infusion followed by electrical cardioversion and discharged with cardiology follow up.

Question
Is cardioversion safe in ED patients presenting with symptomatic atrial fibrillation?

Answer
Yes, the risk of thromboembolism is less than 1% in ED patients who are cardioverted for atrial fibrillation within 48 hours of symptom onset.

References
1. Anderson JL, Halperin JL, Albert NM, et al. "Management of patients with atrial fibrillation (Compilation of 2006 ACCF/AHA/ESC and 2011 ACCF/AHA/HRS Recommendations) a report of the American College of Cardiology/American Heart Association Task Force on Practice Guidelines." *J Am Coll Cardiol.* 2013;61(18):1935–1944.
2. Stiell IG, Clement CM, Perry JJ, et al. Association of the Ottawa Aggresive Protocol with rapid discharge of emergency department patients with recent-onset atrial fibrillation or flutter. *CJEM.* 2010;12(3):181–201.

SECTION 5

ENDOCRINE

Daphne Morrison Ponce

37. ABG vs. VBG in Diabetic Ketoacidosis
38. Bicarbonate Therapy in DKA

ABG VS. VBG IN DIABETIC KETOACIDOSIS

Comparison of Arterial and Venous Blood Gas Values in the Initial Emergency Department Evaluation of Patients with Diabetic Ketoacidosis
Brandenburg MA, Dire DJ. *Ann Emerg Med.* 1998;31(4):459–465

BACKGROUND
Diabetic ketoacidosis (DKA) is responsible for 110,000 hospital admissions annually with a mortality rate up to 10% for patients requiring hospitalization. Effective management of DKA depends on knowing the degree of acidosis. Traditionally this was monitored through arterial sampling which can be painful, technically difficult, and result in vessel injury. At the time of this study, the correlation between venous and arterial pH was well understood but had not been shown to correlate, in the setting of the metabolic derangement that occurs with DKA.

OBJECTIVES
To determine the correlation between venous and arterial pH and venous bicarbonate (HCO_3^-) measurements in DKA patients.

METHODS
Prospective, observational study of patients at a single university teaching hospital in 1996.

Patients
A convenience sample of 44 episodes of DKA (from 38 patients) was analyzed. Inclusion criteria: Arterial pH <7.35 or serum CO_2 <20, serum glucose >250, and positive serum ketones. Participants were excluded if blood samples showed no acidosis.

Intervention Evaluated
ABG and VBG samples were compared for both groups.

Outcomes
The primary outcome was correlation and Bland–Altman analysis of arterial and venous pH, venous HCO_3^- and serum CO_2.

KEY RESULTS
- The mean difference between arterial and venous pH was 0.03 (range 0 to 0.11).
- Ninety-one percent of values fell within the boundaries of agreement.
- One case (2%) differed outside the boundary (0.11); however, this did not alter therapy or management.

STUDY CONCLUSIONS

Peripheral venous pH measurement is a valid and reliable way to measure the degree of acidosis in DKA patients.

COMMENTARY

This study compared ABG and VBG measurement of pH in a patient population that requires frequent pH measuring for both initial diagnosis and monitoring treatment effectiveness. This study lead the movement away from often painful and challenging routine ABGs in favor of a less invasive and just as accurate alternative.

Clinicians should consider obtaining arterial samples in patients if they are working to diagnose concomitant acid–base disorders, as these can be difficult to detect using venous samples.

Question

Can a venous blood gas be used an alternative to an arterial blood gas for pH measurement?

Answer

Yes, the venous blood gas is an accurate initial assessment of acidosis in diabetic ketoacidosis.

CHAPTER 38
BICARBONATE THERAPY IN DKA

Does Bicarbonate Therapy Improve the Management of Severe Diabetic Ketoacidosis?
Viallon A, Zeni F, Lafond P, et al. *Crit Care Med.* 1999;27(12):2690–2693

BACKGROUND
Diabetic ketoacidosis (DKA) has a high mortality rate. Traditional teaching has recommended the use of sodium bicarbonate for patients with pH <7.0. In acidosis, bicarbonate therapy has some theoretically detrimental effects, including worsened hypokalemia, hypocalcemia, CNS, and intracellular acidosis and tissue hypoxia. The balance between the benefits of bicarbonate therapy and these risks had not been investigated prior to this study.

OBJECTIVES
To assess the efficacy of bicarbonate therapy in adult patients with severe DKA (pH <7.10).

METHODS
Retrospective chart review from January 1991 to December 1996.

Patients
Thirty-nine patients with severe DKA as defined by a pH <7.10, plasma glucose concentration >15 mmol/L, and urine ketone concentration >3+.

Intervention Evaluated
Patient charts were retrospectively reviewed and divided into groups based on whether they received sodium bicarbonate infusions. Twenty-four patients received sodium bicarbonate and 15 did not. There was a standard protocol for laboratory tests, intravenous fluid administration, and insulin. The use of sodium bicarbonate was at the discretion of the physician.

Outcomes
The outcomes were biochemical and clinical parameters after 24 hours of admission, the time required for normalization of pH and glycemia, and the time required for clearance of urine ketones.

KEY RESULTS
- No statistical difference existed between the two groups in their biochemical parameters, time to clearance of ketones, or time to normalization of pH and glycemia.

- No significant difference existed between the two groups in their blood potassium; however, the bicarbonate group had a statistically significant higher amount of potassium supplementation.
- There were no episodes of death or hypoglycemia in either group.

STUDY CONCLUSIONS
There is no biochemical or clinical difference between patients with severe DKA (pH 6.90 to 7.10) treated with bicarbonate in addition to standard care.

COMMENTARY
This study showed no benefit to sodium bicarbonate for severe DKA. Although this study was limited by its small size and retrospective nature, the treatment protocols were the same for both study groups. Randomized controlled trials on this topic would be helpful, but such studies are unlikely given the rarity of the disease. Of note, this study only looked at patients with pH 6.90 to 7.10, thus more research is needed for patients with varying degrees of acidemia.

Question
Should ED patients with severe diabetic ketoacidosis (DKA) be treated with bicarbonate?

Answer
No, bicarbonate treatment does not improve biochemical or clinical measures in patients with DKA and a serum pH <7.1.

SECTION 6 INFECTIOUS DISEASE

Kito Lord ■ Ashley Kochanek ■ Jennifer Carnell

39. Early Goal-directed Therapy in Sepsis
40. The PORT Score
41. Steroids in Adult Meningitis
42. Steroids in Pediatric Meningitis
43. Doxycycline in Lyme Disease
44. An Intervention to Decrease Catheter-related Bloodstream Infection
45. Acute Otitis Media and Delayed Antibiotic Treatment
46. Centor Criteria for Strep Throat
47. The Febrile Infant
48. Risk of Serious Bacterial Infection in Febrile Infants with RSV

CHAPTER 39: EARLY GOAL-DIRECTED THERAPY IN SEPSIS

Early Goal-directed Therapy in the Treatment of Severe Sepsis and Septic Shock
Rivers E, Nguyen B, Havstad S, et al. *NEJM.* 2001;345:1368–1377

BACKGROUND
Severe sepsis and septic shock are deadly diseases, with up to 25% mortality. In the late 1990s, small human and animal studies showed potential benefit from early resuscitation to hemodynamic goals to reverse systemic inflammatory response syndrome (SIRS) before deterioration to organ dysfunction and death, mainly in the ICU setting. Rivers et al. postulated that early hemodynamic assessment and aggressive, goal-directed resuscitation of septic patients while still in the ED might improve mortality.

OBJECTIVES
To evaluate the efficacy of early goal-directed therapy (EGDT) in patients with severe sepsis or septic shock in the ED.

METHODS
Prospective, randomized controlled trial conducted in a single American academic ED between 1997 and 2000.

Patients
Two hundred and sixty-three adult patients with at least two SIRS criteria and SBP <90 mm Hg after a 20 to 30 mL/kg crystalloid challenge or a lactate >4 mmol/L. Select exclusion criteria: Patients presenting with noninfectious etiologies of shock (acute coronary syndrome, ischemic or hemorrhagic stroke, drug overdose) or immunosuppression.

Intervention Evaluated
EGDT for 6 hours vs. standard therapy. Both groups received an arterial and central venous catheterization, blood and urine cultures.

EGDT Protocol
500-cc crystalloid boluses targeting central venous pressure (CVP) between 8 and 12 mm Hg. Vasopressors/vasodilators targeting a mean arterial pressure (MAP) of greater than 65 and less than 90. Red cell transfusion to target a hematocrit greater than 30% for central venous oxygen (CVO_2) of less than 70%. If CVO_2 remained less than 70%, dobutamine was given and titrated up unless the MAP was less than 65 or the heart rate was greater than 120 beats per minute. Patients who could not achieve hemodynamic optimization were intubated, mechanically ventilated, and sedated.

Standard therapy was carried out at emergency physician discretion and patients were admitted to the ICU as soon as a bed was available. In both groups, antibiotics were administered at the discretion of the treating physician.

Outcomes
The primary outcome was in-hospital mortality at 28 and 60 days. Secondary outcomes included resuscitation end points at 0 to 6 and 7 to 72 hours and organ dysfunction scores.

KEY RESULTS
- In-hospital mortality was significantly higher in the standard therapy group (46.5% vs. 30.5%) overall and at 28 and 60 days.
- During the initial 6-hour period, 94.9% of patients in the EGDT group achieved CVO_2 >70% vs. 60.2% in the standard group. In the EGDT group 99.2% of patients met the combined therapy goals vs. 86.1% of control group patients.
- During hours 7 to 72 organ dysfunction scores were significantly higher in the standard group indicating more organ dysfunction.
- Risk of sudden cardiovascular collapse as a cause of in-hospital death was higher in the standard group (25 patients vs. 12); multiorgan failure as cause of in-hospital death did not differ significantly between groups.
- The EGDT group received more fluid, blood, inotropic support, and mechanical ventilation in the first 6 hours. The standard therapy group received more fluid, blood, vasopressor support, and mechanical ventilation in the 7- to 72-hour period. Among patients who survived to hospital discharge, standard group patients had longer in-hospital length of stays.

STUDY CONCLUSIONS
EGDT in the ED can improve mortality, severity of organ dysfunction, and hemodynamic parameters in patients presenting with severe sepsis and septic shock.

COMMENTARY
There are high mortality rates and limited, effective clinical interventions for patients with septic shock. In a single center, randomized trial of EGDT vs. standard treatment of patients in early severe sepsis and septic shock, Rivers et al. demonstrate that rapid diagnosis and initiation of therapy in the ED are paramount to improving survival. This study made the term EGDT standard lexicon across EDs in the United States and introduced the potential effectiveness of protocolized, target driven approaches to improving outcomes. These findings should be interpreted with some caution as the interventions and targets selected were based on small studies and expert consensus, and not rigorously conducted trails of each element. Subsequent research has shown certain elements to be very valuable and others lacking clear benefit,[1-4] and presented new and improved monitoring parameters[5,6] and interventions.[7,8] EGDT continues to serve as the basis for the international Surviving Sepsis Campaign, critical care clinical practice guidelines, and national quality measures seeking to improve mortality for this deadly disease.[9]

Question

Does early goal-directed therapy improve outcomes in septic ED patients?

Answer

Yes, early goal-directed therapy reduces mortality by establishing a protocol for early recognition and resuscitation of patients in severe sepsis and septic shock.[9]

References

1. Parsons EC, Hough CL, Seymour CW, et al. Red blood cell transfusion and outcomes in patients with acute lung injury, sepsis and shock. *Crit Care.* 2011;15(5):R221.
2. Shorr AF, Jackson WL, Kelly KM, et al. Transfusion practice and blood stream infections in critically ill patients. *Chest.* 2005;127:1722–1728.
3. Marik PE, Corwin HL. Efficacy of red blood cell transfusion in the critically ill: A systematic review of the literature. *Crit Care Med.* 2008;36:2667–2674.
4. The ProCESS Investigators. A Randomized Trial of Protocol-Based Care for Early Septic Shock. *NEJM.* 2014;370(18):1683–1693.
5. Jones AE, Shapiro NI, Trzeciak S, et al. Lactate clearance vs. central venous oxygen saturation as goals of early sepsis therapy: A randomized clinical trial. *JAMA.* 2010;303:739–746.
6. Nguyen HB, Loomba M, Yang JJ, et al. Early lactate clearance is associated with biomarkers of inflammation, coagulation, apoptosis, organ dysfunction and mortality in severe sepsis and septic shock. *J Inflam.* 2010;7:6.
7. Russell JA1, Walley KR, Singer J, et al. Vasopressin versus norepinephrine infusion in patients with septic shock. *NEJM.* 2008;358(9):877–887.
8. De Backer D, Biston P, Devriendt J, et al. Comparison of dopamine and norepinephrine in the treatment of shock. *N Engl J Med.* 2010;362:779–789.
9. Dellinger RP, Levy MM, Rhodes A, et al. Surviving Sepsis Campaign: International guidelines for management of severe sepsis and septic shock, 2012. *Intensive Care Med.* 2013;39(2):165–228.

CHAPTER 40: THE PORT SCORE

A Prediction Rule to Identify Low-risk Patients with Community-acquired Pneumonia
Fine MJ, Auble TE, Yealy DM, et al. *N Engl J Med.* 1997;336(4):243–250

BACKGROUND
At the time of this study, pneumonia was the eighth leading cause of death in the United States leading to over 600,000 hospital admissions annually. Aggregate hospitalization costs for the disease approached $4 billion per year. Significant geographic variation in the rate of hospitalization of patients with community-acquired pneumonia (CAP) suggested that inconsistent criteria were being used to determine patients' need for hospitalization. There was no accurate, objective model for prognosis in CAP that could guide the decision to hospitalize patients.

OBJECTIVES
To create a prediction rule using easily obtained variables that accurately identifies patients with CAP who are at low risk for death and thereby help physicians better identify patients who can be safely discharged.

METHODS
Observational cohort study, including retrospective rule derivation, and prospective rule validation, at 78 hospitals across 23 states between 1989 and 1991.

Participants
Derivation cohort: 14,199 adult patients from the 1989 MedisGroup database with a principal diagnosis of pneumonia according to ICD-9 code. Select exclusion criteria: HIV and hospitalization within 7 days of presentation.

Validation cohort: 38,039 patients from the 1991 MedisGroup database with a principal diagnosis of pneumonia, as well as the Pneumonia PORT study cohort of 2,287 patients.

Intervention Evaluated
The prediction rule derived from the retrospective cohort was validated using the 1991 MedisGroup database, and then was prospectively applied to the Pneumonia PORT study cohort.

Outcomes
The primary outcome was 30-day mortality.

KEY RESULTS
- The final two-step prediction rule and point scoring system was created from the tested variables.

- Eighteen factors were independently associated with 30-day mortality: Age >50, chronic congestive heart failure, liver disease, kidney disease, cerebrovascular disease, and neoplastic disease, and examination findings of altered mental status, heart rate >125, respiratory rate >30, systolic blood pressure <90, and temperature <35 or >40, and blood urea nitrogen (BUN) >30, glucose >250, hematocrit <31%, sodium <130, partial pressure of arterial oxygen <60 mm Hg, arterial pH <7.35, and pleural effusion were independently associated with 30-day mortality.
- Point scores were summed and used to divide patients into five classes. Class I had no step one risk factors and had a mortality risk of 0.1% in all cohorts. Class II had a mortality risk of <1%, class III <4%, class IV 4% to 10%, and class V >10%.

STUDY CONCLUSIONS

The PORT Score prediction rule accurately identifies patients with CAP who are at low risk for death within 30 days using readily available ED data.

COMMENTARY

This study provides a simple means of identifying low-risk patients with CAP using readily available clinical data derived and validated in diverse, large cohorts both retrospectively and prospectively. It is especially useful in the case of class I patients, who can be designated very low risk using only demographic, history and physical examination data without laboratories or radiography and sent home. Clinician should exercise some caution in applying the PORT score as the clinical decision rule does not include some frequently important variables for clinical decision making including pulse oximetry, unstable psychosocial situations, substance abuse, rare comorbid conditions, and immunosuppression which could alter patient's risk of death. Since the PORT score established the effectiveness of risk stratification in CAP, a new, streamlined CAP risk stratification score the CURB-65 (confusion, uremia >19 mg/dL, respiratory rate >30, systolic blood pressure <90, and age >65) was created and validated by Lim et al.[1] Both the PORT and CURB-65 scores have become standard of care in the Infectious Disease Society of America CAP guidelines.[2]

Question

Can the PORT score differentiate between pneumonia patients at a high or low risk of death?

Answer

Yes, patients with Class I to Class III scores are at low risk of mortality and should be considered for outpatient care, while PORT Class IV patients have a high risk of mortality and require hospitalization.

Table 40.1 The Port Score: Pneumonia Severity Index for Community Acquired Pneumonia

Step 1. Is the patient at low risk (class I) based on the history and physical examination and not a resident of a nursing home? • Age 50 yr or younger and • None of the coexisting conditions or physical examination findings listed in step 2		
No: Go to step 2. Yes: Outpatient treatment is recommended.		
Step 2. Calculate risk score for classes II to V.		
Patient Characteristics	**Points Assigned**	**Patient's Points**
Demographic factors		
Age (in years)		
Males	Age	_____
Females	Age – 10	_____
Nursing home resident	+10	_____
Coexisting conditions		
Neoplastic disease	+30	_____
Liver disease	+20	_____
Congestive heart failure	+10	_____
Cerebrovascular disease	+10	_____
Renal disease	+10	_____
Initial physical examination findings		
Altered mental status	+20	_____
Respiratory rate ≥30 breaths per minute	+20	_____
Systolic blood pressure <90 mm Hg	+20	_____
Temperature <35°C (95°F) or ≥40°C (104°F)	+15	_____
Pulse ≥125 beats per minute	+10	_____
Initial laboratory findings (score zero if not tested)		
pH <7.35	+30	_____
Blood urea nitrogen >30 mg per dL (10.5 mmol per L)	+20	_____
Sodium <130 mEq per L (130 mmol per L)	+20	_____
Glucose ≥250 mg per dL (13.9 mmol per L)	+10	_____
Hematocrit <30 percent (0.30)	+10	_____

(continued)

Arterial PO$_2$ <60 mm Hg or O$_2$ saturation <90 percent	+10	
Pleural effusion	+10	
Total score (sum of patient's points)		

30-day Mortality Data by Risk Class

Total Score	Risk Class	Recommended Site of Treatment	Mortality Range Observed in Validation Cohorts (%)
None (see step 1)	I	Outpatient	0.1
≤70	II	Outpatient	0.6
71–90	III	Outpatient	0.9–2.8
91–130	IV	Inpatient	8.2–9.3
>130	V	Inpatient	27–29.2

References
1. Lim WS, van der Eerden MM, Laing R, et al. Defining community acquired pneumonia severity on presentation to hospital: An international derivation and validation study. *Thorax.* 2003;58(5):377–382.
2. Aujesky D, Auble TE, Yealy DM, et al. Prospective comparison of three validated prediction rules for prognosis in community-acquired pneumonia. *Am J Med.* 2005;118(4):384–392.

CHAPTER 41: STEROIDS IN ADULT MENINGITIS

Dexamethasone in adults with bacterial meningitis
de Gans J, van de Beek D, European Dexamethasone in Adulthood Bacterial Meningitis Study Investigators. *N Engl J Med.* 2002;347(20):1549–1556

BACKGROUND
Acute bacterial meningitis carries high morbidity and mortality, thought to be partly a result of inflammation in the CNS secondary to the bacteriolytic effect of appropriate antibiotic treatment. Previous small, nonrandomized studies in adults, children, and animal models suggested that adjuvant treatment with corticosteroids might benefit adults with bacterial meningitis by decesing this inflammatory response; however, no randomized trial had been done.

OBJECTIVES
To evaluate whether adjunctive dexamethasone treatment improves outcomes in adult patients with bacterial meningitis.

METHODS
Multicenter, prospective, randomized, double-blind trial in the Netherlands between June 1993 and December 2001. Patients were randomized to dexamethasone or placebo. All patients were initially treated with amoxicillin with changes permitted at the discretion of the treating physician.

Participants
Three hundred and one patients, >17 years old, with suspected meningitis in combination with cloudy Cerebral Spinal Fluid (CSF), CSF leukocyte count >1,000/mm^3, or CSF with bacteria on Gram stain. Select exclusion criteria: Antibiotics in the previous 48 hours, neurosurgery, recent head trauma, or peptic ulcer disease.

Intervention Evaluated
Dexamethasone 10 mg every 6 hours, beginning at the time of antibiotic initiation and continued for 4 days, compared to placebo.

Outcomes
The primary outcome was Glasgow Outcome Scale, a 1 to 5 assessment of neurologic functional status that broadly categorizes patients as (1) dead, (2) vegetative, (3) severely impaired, (4) able to live independently but not return to work, and (5) able to return to work, at 8 weeks after randomization. Secondary outcomes were death, focal neurologic abnormalities, hearing loss, clinically relevant gastrointestinal bleeding, or infection.

KEY RESULTS
- At 8 weeks more patients in the placebo group had unfavorable outcomes, as defined by a Glasgow Outcome Scale <5, than in the dexamethasone group (25% vs. 15%).
- Patients treated with dexamethasone had lower mortality (7% vs. 15%).
- The lower mortality in the dexamethasone group did not result in an increased rate of severe neurologic sequelae.
- Overall, dexamethasone did not increase risk of adverse events.

STUDY CONCLUSIONS
Early treatment with dexamethasone improves neurologic outcome and reduces risk of death in adult patients with acute bacterial meningitis.

COMMENTARY
This was the first multicenter, double-blinded, placebo-controlled trial of steroids in adults with acute bacterial meningitis and demonstrated a clear benefit from steroids in a reasonably generalizable population of healthy adults. This study spurred subsequent research on steroid use in adult and pediatric meningitis which have shown less hearing loss and fewer neurologic sequelae, but did not reproduce the mortality benefit.[1] Given the mortality and functional outcomes benefit and low risk seen in this and subsequent studies, the Infectious Disease Society of America (IDSA) guidelines currently recommend adjunctive dexamethasone in all adults with suspected acute bacterial meningitis and in children on a case-by-case basis.

Question
Do steroids improve outcomes in adults with acute bacterial meningitis?

Answer
Yes, early dexamethasone treatment in addition to early, appropriate antibiotics reduces the risk of death and adverse neurologic outcomes in adults with suspected meningitis.

Reference
1. Brouwer MC, McIntyre P, de Gans J, Prasad K, van de Beek D. Corticosteroids for acute bacterial meningitis. *Cochrane Database Syst Rev.* 2010;(9):CD004405.

CHAPTER 42: STEROIDS IN PEDIATRIC MENINGITIS

The Beneficial Effects of Early Dexamethasone Administration in Infants and Children with Bacterial Meningitis
Odio CM, Faingezicht I, Paris M, et al. *N Engl J Med.* 1991;324(22):1525–1531

BACKGROUND
Bacterial meningitis is a life-threatening illness with high neurologic morbidity. Animal models showed an increase in inflammatory markers after administration of antibiotics that was coincident with increases in cell wall products from the destroyed bacteria. This immune response was thought to worsen outcomes and some prior studies had demonstrated potential benefit with dexamethasone use in adult patients if given prior to administration of antibiotics. At the time of this study no experimental study had been conducted in children.

OBJECTIVES
To determine the clinical effect of dexamethasone in children with bacterial meningitis.

METHODS
Randomized, placebo-controlled, double-blinded study conducted in a single center in Costa Rica.

Patients
One hundred and one infants and children age 6 weeks to 13 years diagnosed with bacterial meningitis. Approximately 80% were younger than 2 years and 90% younger than 5 years.

Intervention Evaluated
Administration of dexamethasone before cefotaxime (n = 52) vs. placebo and cefotaxime (n = 49). The patients and evaluators were blinded to the treatment modality. Patient allotted to each group had cerebrospinal fluid (CSF) pressures, lactate, tumor necrosis factor α (TNF-alpha), and platelet-activating factor (PAF) measured. Patients with open fontanelles underwent ultrasonography and those with closed fontanelles underwent computed tomographic scanning.

Outcomes
The primary outcome was degree of meningeal inflammation, characterized by cerebral pressure and inflammatory markers. The secondary outcome was improved outcome of the disease evaluated by neurologic sequelae and hearing function.

KEY RESULTS
- Inflammatory markers, such as TNF-alpha, leukocyte concentration, and protein were all significantly reduced at 12 hours in the dexamethasone group when compared to placebo.
- Opening CSF pressures were lower in the dexamethasone group compared to the placebo (166 ± 65 vs. 199 ± 58); however, this lost statistical significance after 12 hours.
- The dexamethasone group had less neurologic sequelae at 5 to 25 months than the placebo group. There was a relative risk of 3.8.
- The dexamethasone group had fewer days of fever (1.3 ± 1.2 vs. 4.3 ± 2.5 days).

STUDY CONCLUSIONS
Dexamethasone improves outcomes in infants and children with bacterial meningitis when administered before initiation of cefotaxime therapy.

COMMENTARY
Bacterial meningitis is a life-threatening illness that has significant mortality and morbidity. There had been some evidence to suggest a reduction in mortality and improved neurologic outcomes in adults; however, like for many acute care interventions, there was a paucity of evidence in children. The authors were able to demonstrate an initial reduction in inflammatory markers in the CSF but no change in mortality at 48 hours. Although they were unable to find a difference in audiologic outcomes, a composite endpoint of audiologic and neurologic sequelae reached clinical significance at 5 to 25 months after discharge. As a result, the study conclusions should be interpreted with some caution as the secondary outcome was not the intent of this study and the pathophysiologic linkage between a single dose of steroids and long-term outcomes is tenable. In addition, this study did not include neonates. Also note, with the advent of newer vaccinations for *Haemophilus influenzae* type b, which represented 78% of the bacterial infections in this study, bacterial meningitis of this etiology has become a rare disease which may limit the generalizability of these findings. Despite these limitations, this study laid the groundwork for current practice, reflecting the Infectious Disease Society of America recommendations, to administer dexamethasone prior to antibiotics in children with acute bacterial meningitis.

Question
Do steroids improve outcomes in infants and children with bacterial meningitis?

Answer
Yes, when given 15 to 20 minutes prior to administration of antibiotics, dexamethasone may reduce overall neurologic sequelae in *Haemophilus influenzae* type b bacterial meningitis.

CHAPTER 43
DOXYCYCLINE IN LYME DISEASE

Prophylaxis with Single-dose Doxycycline for the Prevention of Lyme Disease after an Ixodes Scapularis Tick Bite
Nadelman RB, Nowakowski J, Fish D, et al. *N Engl J Med.* 2001;345(2):79–84

BACKGROUND
Lyme disease (*Borrelia burgdorferi*) is transmitted by the bite of the *Ixodes scapularis* tick and causes significant morbidity in endemic regions. Prior research into other spirochete infections such as syphilis and leptospirosis suggested benefit in prophylactic antimicrobial treatment of incubating spirochete infections. At the time of this study, it was unknown whether antimicrobial prophylaxis after an *I. scapularis* tick bite would prevent Lyme disease.

OBJECTIVES
To determine if primary prophylaxis with a single dose of doxycycline would prevent Lyme disease after an *I. scapularis* tick bite.

METHODS
Randomized, double-blind, placebo-controlled trial at a single academic medical center in Westchester County, NY between May 1987 and December 1996.

Patients
Four hundred and eighty-two patients, >12 years old, residing in a Lyme hyperendemic area who had been bitten by an *I. scapularis* tick and had removed the tick from their body within 72 hours. Tick species and duration of attachment were confirmed by a medical entomologist. Subjects were excluded if they could not provide the tick, had evidence of Lyme infection, and had recently received antibiotics effective against *B. burgdorferi* or Lyme vaccination.

Intervention Evaluated
A single dose of 200 mg of oral doxycycline administered within 72 hours of an *I. scapularis* tick bite.

Outcomes
The primary outcome was development of erythema migrans at the site of the tick bite. Secondary outcomes included erythema migrans at a site distinct from the initial tick bite and positive *B. burgdorferi* IgM serum antibodies.

KEY RESULTS
- Single-dose doxycycline was found to have an 87% efficacy: 1 out of 235 subjects in the doxycycline group and 8 out of 247 in the placebo group developed erythema migrans.
- Nausea and vomiting were more common in the doxycycline group but were self limited and no serious adverse effects were observed.

STUDY CONCLUSIONS
A single dose of 200 mg of doxycycline given within 72 hours after an *I. scapularis* tick bite can prevent the development of Lyme disease.

COMMENTARY
Lyme disease is a highly prevalent illness in hyperendemic regions with hundreds of thousands of patients exposed to tick bites and the potentially morbid effects untreated Lyme disease. This double-blinded, placebo-control trial demonstrated that an inexpensive, convenient single-dose prophylactic regimen could effectively prevent Lyme disease. The study is most applicable to patients in hyperendemic Lyme regions, since the incidence of Lyme disease per tick bitten patient will be greater and the number needed to treat will be smaller (Lyme infection rates in the hyperendemic study population were only 3% in the untreated group). In addition, no subjects in the study developed any of the more severe, extracutaneous manifestations of Lyme disease such as Bell palsy, heart block, meningeal signs, thus it is unclear if single-dose doxycycline provides prophylaxis against these more severe consequences of Lyme disease. Despite these limitations, the current Infectious Disease Society of America (IDSA) guidelines selectively recommend offering doxycycline to adult patients and children >8 years of age for tick bites of greater than 36-hour attachment in hyperendemic regions.

Question
Can antibiotics prevent the development of Lyme disease?

Answer
Yes, a one-time dose of doxycycline within 72 hours of a tick bite can effectively prevent erythema migrans in hyperendemic regions.

CHAPTER 44
AN INTERVENTION TO DECREASE CATHETER-RELATED BLOODSTREAM INFECTION

An Intervention to Decrease Catheter-related Bloodstream Infections in the ICU
Pronovost P, Needham D, Berenholtz S, et al. *N Engl J Med.* 2006;355(26):2725–2732

BACKGROUND
Central line-associated bloodstream infections (CLABSI) were estimated to cause 80,000 cases of central line-associated infections and as many as 28,000 deaths in the United States. Each catheter-related infection can cost as much as $11,971 to $54,000, per infection. At the time of this study, it was unclear how many of these infections were preventable. It was theorized that changes in the placement and management of central catheters could potentially save thousands of lives and reduce hospital stays; however, no study had broadly demonstrated optimal practices to achieve this goal.

OBJECTIVES
To implement an intervention to reduce the incidence of CLABSI in intensive care units (ICUs).

METHODS
Prospective observational study at 67 hospitals, including 108 ICUs in Michigan between March 2004 and September 2005.

Patients
375,757 catheter days across 103 ICUs. Inclusion criteria: Central venous catheters (CVCs), including PICC lines, in patients in an ICU bed. Multiple lines in one patient were counted as 1 catheter day.

Intervention Evaluated
Standard implementation of five CDC recommended guidelines deemed to have the highest impact on infection control and the lowest barriers to implementation including, (1) hand washing, (2) full-barrier precautions, (3) cleaning skin with chlorhexidine, (4) avoiding femoral site, and (5) removing unnecessary catheters. To accomplish this task, the authors designated team leaders and provided education. Central lines were accompanied with checklist and later chlorhexidine. During the procedure, providers were stopped for nonadherence to central line protocol. Monthly feedback and education was given to ICU staff.

Outcomes
Quarterly rate of CLABSI, as defined by the National Nosocomial Infection Surveillance System.

KEY RESULTS
- There was a mean CLABSI reduction from 7.7 to 1.4 per 1,000 catheter days.
- There was a mean CLABSI reduction from 2.7 to 0 per 1,000 catheter das in 3 months after implementation.
- At 18 months the number CLABSI remained at 0 (mean, 1.4).
- Incident ratios showed decrease in CLABSI from 0.62 at 0 to 3 months to 0.34 at 16 to 18 months.
- Teaching hospitals showed an incidence ratio that did not show statistical significance with a value of 1.34.

STUDY CONCLUSIONS
Implementation of an evidence-based intervention for CLABSI can significantly reduce the rate of infections and sustain these results.

COMMENTARY
Placement of a central line can be a life-saving procedure; however, it also can lead to significant mortality and morbidity. To demonstrate the effectiveness of widely adopting safe health care practices, this study was designed as part of a real-world quality improvement collaborative directed at reducing the number of bloodstream infections related to central venous catheters in the ICU. By using the CDC guidelines related to CVC practices, in addition to education, standardized definitions of CVC infections, and daily discussions on rounds, the study showed a median reductions from 2.7 to 0 per 1,000 catheter days and sustained these results for 15 months across an extremely large sample of hospitals. These results show the potential for improving infection prevention in high-risk, critically ill patients who are often in the ED; however, these findings may not be generalizable to central lines placed under crowded, emergent, or other conditions that make following national patient safety guidelines challenging. Despite these hurdles, the development of checklists and comprehensive central venous catheter protocols have been developed for ED and hospital-wide use nationally as all providers seek to replicate this zero infection rate outcome.

Question
Do specific provider practices reduce the likelihood of catheter-related bloodstream infections?

Answer
Yes, use of a standard checklist for central venous line placement can reduce the rate of bloodstream infections to near zero.

ACUTE OTITIS MEDIA AND DELAYED ANTIBIOTIC TREATMENT

CHAPTER 45

Wait-and-see Prescription for the Treatment of Acute Otitis Media: A Randomized Controlled Trial

Spiro DM, Tay KY, Arnold DH, Dziura JD, Baker MD, Shapiro ED. *JAMA*. 2006;296(10):1235–1241.

BACKGROUND

Acute otitis media (AOM) is one of the most frequent pediatric ED diagnoses leading to an estimated 15 million antibiotic prescriptions a year. Usually triggered by a viral illness, the middle ear effusions of AOM often contain bacteria isolates and can lead to complications, such as mastoiditis. Despite this, a large number of AOM will resolve spontaneously. Prior studies had specifically excluded children with severe otitis media and those with fevers and were convenience samples leaving uncertainty regarding how effective an antibiotic-optional approach would work. Given the complications associated with antibiotic use (including allergy, bacterial resistance, and diarrhea), it was posited that the number of infections treated with antibiotics could be reduced using a wait-and-see approach.

OBJECTIVES

To determine whether treatment of AOM using a wait-and-see prescription approach would reduce the use of antibiotics and to evaluate the impact of this intervention on clinical symptoms and adverse outcomes.

METHODS

Randomized control trial at a single academic urban pediatric ED between 2004 and 2005.

Patients

Two hundred and eighty-three patients, aged 6 months to 12 years, determined by the treating physician to have AOM. Select exclusion criteria (n = 493): Patients admitted to the hospital, concurrent bacterial infection, antibiotics in the last 7 days, myringotomy tubes, or perforated tympanic membrane or uncertain access to medical care.

Intervention Evaluated

Patients were randomized to the wait-and-see prescription or standard prescription group. The wait-and-see prescription group was given an antibiotic prescription and instructed not to fill this unless the child did not improve within 48 hours. The standard prescription group was given antibiotics and told to fill the prescription following the ED visit. Both groups received ibuprofen and otic analgesic.

Outcomes

The primary outcome was the ratio of each group that filled the antibiotic prescription. The secondary outcomes included clinical course of the illness, adverse effects of medications, days of school missed, unscheduled medical visits, and comfort of parents managing AOM.

KEY RESULTS
- Significantly less patients in the wait-and-see prescription group filled their prescriptions as compared to the standard prescription group (13% vs. 62%).
- There was no statistical difference between fever, otalgia, or unscheduled medical care on follow-up.
- Fever and otalgia were associated with filling the prescription in the wait-and-see group.

STUDY CONCLUSIONS
Wait-and-see-prescription approach to patients with AOM can lead to a reduction of antibiotic use.

COMMENTARY
With increasing bacterial resistance and heightened attention to the risk of allergic reactions, this study challenged the standard practice of routine prescriptions for antibiotics for AOM. Prior studies that examined a similar wait-and-see-prescription approach were neither conducted in an ED setting nor did they systematically treat otalgia and fever. This study allowed for symptomatic treatment, which is an important component in the outpatient management of AOM. Furthermore, the study included structured, prospective follow-up so that meaningful patient-oriented outcomes, such as unscheduled medical care of missed school days, could be assessed. In addition to showing equivalent clinical outcomes in the wait-and-see group, the study confirmed fears related to antibiotic overprescribing as the group using immediate antibiotics had almost three times the rate of diarrhea as the wait-and-see-prescription group (wait-and-see prescription 8% vs. standard prescription 23%). Broad acceptance of this study's findings helped update the American Academy of Pediatrics 2013 guidelines that support the wait-and-see-prescription approach when good follow-up is available in the ED.

Question
Does acute otitis media in children always warrant immediate antibiotic therapy?

Answer
No, the wait-and-see approach appears to be a safe and viable option to reduce the risk and harm associated with antibiotic use in children.

CHAPTER 46
CENTOR CRITERIA FOR STREP THROAT

The Diagnosis of Strep Throat in Adults in the Emergency Room
Centor RM, Witherspoon JM, Dalton HP, Brody CE, Link K. *Med Decis Making.* 1981;1(3):239–246

BACKGROUND
Sore throat is a common ED presentation, with over 11 million cases of pharyngitis in US EDs and ambulatory clinics annually. Although Group A beta-hemolytic streptococcus (GAS) is the most common bacterial etiology of pharyngitis, the vast majority of cases are viral (80% to 95% in adults, 70% to 85% in children). Prior to this study, no simple set of criteria existed to accurately evaluate the likelihood that a patient with sore throat would have a positive culture based on history and physical examination findings, and thus there was no simple way for clinicians to predict which patients were unlikely to benefit from antibiotic treatment for GAS pharyngitis.

OBJECTIVES
To identify the prevalence of GAS in adults presenting with sore throat to an urban ED and to develop a model to determine the likelihood of bacterial pharyngitis.

METHODS
Prospective, observational study in an urban ED in 1980.

Participants
Two hundred and eighty-six consecutive patients, >15 years old, with sore throat. Select exclusion criteria: Patients whose throat cultures grew non-GAS (predominantly Groups B, C, and G). Control group was made up of 25 patients and employees aged 16 to 35 with no upper respiratory symptoms.

Interventions
Each study subject underwent throat culture. For all cultures positive for GAS, the specific type of beta streptococcus was determined using a rapid latex test.

Outcomes
Based on culture results and clinical information, models were constructed, using logistic regression analysis, for both a positive culture and a resident's belief that the patient would have a positive culture.

KEY RESULTS
- Seventeen percent of throat cultures from study subjects with sore throat grew GAS. None of the cultures from the control group (without respiratory symptoms) grew GAS.

- The model derived for a positive culture included four variables: (1) tonsillar exudates, (2) swollen tender anterior cervical nodes, (3) lack of a cough, and (4) fever history.
- The probability of a positive culture was predicted by the number of variables present in the patient: 4/4 = 55.7%, 3/4 = 30.1% to 34.1%, 2/4 = 14.1% to 16.6%, 1/4 = 6% to 6.9%, 0/4 = 2.5% probability of a positive culture.
- A resident's guess demonstrated 0.72 sensitivity and 0.76 specificity in predicting a positive throat culture.

STUDY CONCLUSIONS

A simple model that includes four variables can be used to predict the probability of a positive throat culture for GAS and can help to guide clinical management.

COMMENTARY

This study was designed to identify a simple set of variables that can be used to predict the probability of a positive throat culture for GAS in adults with sore throat. Prior studies used complex models to predict a positive culture but those models were difficult to remember and, therefore, of limited usefulness in the clinical setting. The four Centor criteria are easy to remember and use when evaluating adult patients with sore throat. When patients have none or only one of the Centor criteria, their probability of having a throat culture positive for GAS is very low; therefore, clinicians may feel more confident in their decision to not prescribe antibiotics before culture results are available. Conversely, even when patients with sore throat are positive for all four of the Centor criteria, the probability that the throat culture will be positive for GAS is only 55.7%. Therefore, prescribing antibiotics based on Centor criteria positivity would lead to treatment of a large number of patients who do not have streptococcal pharyngitis. In the adult age group, where GAS pharyngitis is rare and the feared sequelae of rheumatic fever and carditis are even more rare, the individual and public health risks of overprescribing antibiotics would outweigh the risks of not treating a patient. In 2000, a modified Centor criterion[1] was validated with an additional point for age <15 years which greatly improved sensitivity and specificity (85% and 92%), and is now widely used in clinical practice.

Question

Is a clinical history and physical examination sufficient to make treatment decision for a patient with a sore throat?

Answer

Yes, the presence or absence of four clinical variables predicts the probability of a positive throat culture for Group A beta-hemolytic streptococcus and can guide antibiotic prescribing decisions.

Reference

1. McIsaac WJ, Kellner JD, Aufricht P, et al. Empirical Validation of Guidelines for the Management of Pharyngitis in Children and Adults. *JAMA*. 2004;291(13):1587–1595.

CHAPTER 47 THE FEBRILE INFANT

Outpatient Treatment of Febrile Infants 28 to 89 Days of Age With Intramuscular Administration of Ceftriaxone
Baskin MN, O'Rourke EJ, Fleisher GR. *J Pediatr.* 1992:120(1):22–27

Outpatient Management Without Antibiotics of Fever in Selected Infants
Baker MD, Bell LM, Avner JR. *N Engl J Med.* 1993;329(20):1437–1441

Febrile Infants at Low Risk for Serious Bacterial Infection–An Appraisal of the Rochester Criteria and Implications for Management. Febrile Infant Collaborative Study Group
Jaskiewicz, JA, McCarthy CA, Richardson AC, et al. *Pediatrics.* 1994;94:(3):390–396

BACKGROUND

The management of a febrile infant less than 3 months of age has been an area of debate for decades. At times, relatively healthy-looking infants have occult bacteremia presenting a diagnostic challenge to the physician. Prior to these studies, it was common practice to admit all febrile infants under 90 days for close observation. No studies had yet evaluated the role of risk stratification to identify low-risk febrile infants, empiric antibiotics, and outpatient management.

OBJECTIVES

The *Boston* group attempted to determine whether it was safe to discharge infants with a low risk of occult bacteremia home after intramuscular ceftriaxone (IM CTX). The *Philadelphia* group tried to evaluate the efficacy of managing fever in young infants without empiric antibiotics or routine hospitalization and to assess the savings associated with this approach. The *Rochester* group assessed whether infants without a serious bacterial infection (SBI) could be identified by a set of criteria.

COMMENTARY

These studies continue to be the foundation for the management of febrile infants and are the basis of many clinical guidelines found in pediatrics, family medicine, and emergency medicine. Each attempts to identify infants that are low risk and who can be managed as outpatients either with or without antibiotics. Each set of criteria has limitations—the Boston criteria treat many patients with antibiotics that may not need them. The Philadelphia criteria require a large amount of invasive testing before an infant is determined to be safe to send home, and the Rochester criteria do not include LP as part of the criteria and with a 1% SBI rate in the low-risk group. In addition, the Philadelphia and Boston criteria did not include neonates and should no the used in this patient population. The 2003 ACEP clinical guideline suggest all neonates be presumed to have an SBI. Adherence to the guidelines that these studies inform has been shown to be variable in a number of studies and surveys as admissions decisions may often be driven by variable patient and provider risk tolerance as well as social concerns. However, all studies show that safe outpatient management is possible and that routine admission of all febrile infants is unnecessary.

	Boston	Philadelphia	Rochester
Methods	Single center prospective consecutive cohort at an urban pediatric ED from 1987 to 1990	Prospective randomized single center study at an urban, pediatric ED from 1987 to 1992	Three prospective studies, two at Rochester Hospital and one data set in multicenter EDs from 1984 to 1992
Participants	503 febrile infants aged 28–89 days with: (1) T >38°C rectal or parent reported; (2) Well appearing, normal examination and vital signs; (3) No evidence of ear, soft tissue, joint, or bone infection; (4) Care giver available by telephone; (5) No vaccination or antibiotics 48 hours prior; (6) CSF WBC <10/µL; (7) Peripheral leukocyte <20,000/µL; (8) UA <10 leukocytes/hpf; (9) No CXR infiltrate, if obtained	747 consecutive infants 29–56 d of age with: (1) T >38.2; (2) Infant Observation Score ≤10; (3) Peripheral WBC <15,000/cc; (4) Bandemia to neutrophil ratio <0.2; (5) Urinalysis <10 WBC/hpf and few or no bacteria; (6) CSF <8 WBC/µL; (6) No CXR infiltrate, if ordered	1,057 infants <60 days of age with T >38°C. Rochester criteria were then used to identify infants at low risk of SBI: (1) Infant appears well; (2) Infant has been previously healthy; (3) No evidence of soft tissue, bone, joint, or ear infection; (4) Normal laboratory values (WBC count 5,000 to 15,000/cc, bandemia <1,500/cc, ≤10 WBC/hpf on spun urine, and ≤5 WBC/hpf on stool smear)
Intervention	Blood, urine, and CSF cultures sent, 50 mg/kg of IM CTX, and discharged home. Return within 24 h for reevaluation and second dose of IM CTX. Patients were followed at 48 hours and 7 days.	All had LP, CBC, UA, CXR, and stool studies if history diarrhea. Those who did not meet criteria ($n = 460$) received antibiotics and admission. Those who met inclusion criteria were randomized to (1) inpatient observation no antibiotics ($n = 139$) or (2) outpatient observation no antibiotics ($n = 148$). Patients reevaluated in person at 24 and 48 h by attending physicians in the ED.	All had LP, CBC, UA, CXR when indicated, and cultures of stool, blood, urine, and CSF. Patients divided into low risk ($n = 437$) and not low risk ($n = 511$) over three studies using the Rochester criteria.

(continued)

	Boston	Philadelphia	Rochester
Outcomes	Primary—number of infants discharged home later determined to have an SBI after IM CTX. SBI defined as bacteria growth in cultures of blood, CSF, urine, or stool. Secondary outcome—comparison with Rochester Criteria.	Primary—number of SBI and cost. SBI defined as bacterial growth in blood, CSF, urine, or stool cultures, pneumonia, aseptic meningitis, or cellulitis.	Primary outcome—ability of the Rochester criteria to identify infants unlikely to have an SBI, defined as bacterial growth in blood, CSF, urine or evidence of osteomyelitis, suppurative arthritis, cellullitis, gastroenteritis or pneumonia. Secondary outcome—determine whether modifications to the Rochester criteria should be evaluated further.
Key Results	• 5.4% met SBI criteria and 94.6% did not. • 1.7% found to have occult bacteremia. • UTI without bacteremia (1.6%) and bacterial gastroenteritis without bacteremia (10%) were the other two causes of SBI. • 23 infants who did not meet SBI criteria were admitted, but only two appeared ill. • 13 of the 25 infants of the SBI group would have been identified as high risk by the Rochester criteria (sensitivity = 0.52). • ~1,167 hospital days were eliminated during the 39 month study	• Sensitivity was 98% and negative predictive value was 100%. • One patient assigned to outpatient group was admitted but determined not to have SBI, and two of the inpatient-observation group were found to have SBI. • Additional criteria of immunodeficiency and band to neutrophil ratio <0.2 increased NPV to 100%. • Average charges: Inpatient antibiotics: $5,532. Inpatient observation: $3,311. Outpatient observation: $784. • Outpatient observation was $2,500 cheaper than inpatient observation.	• Overall rate of SBI was 7%. • SBI occurred in 1% of low-risk infants. All five had variable antimicrobial intervention and follow-up but all did well. • SBI occurred in 12.3% of infants not in the low-risk group. • NPV was 98.9% for any SBI. • NPV was 99.5% for bacteremia. • Eighty-eight percent of infants who did not meet low-risk criteria also did not have SBI.
Study Conclusions	Outpatient management with IM CTX, after a full evaluation for sepsis and with adherence to a strict follow-up protocol is a safe alternative to hospital admission.	The Philadelphia protocol can safely identify a group of febrile infants who are at low risk for SBI and can be safely managed at home without antibiotics.	This data confirms the ability of low-risk criteria to identify infants unlikely to have SBI. Infants and neonates who meet the low-risk criteria can be carefully observed without administering antibiotics.

T: Temperature, WBC: White blood cell count, CSF: Cerebral spinal fluid, UA: urinalaysis, CXR: chest xray, CTX: Ceftriaxone, LP: Lumbar puncture.

Question

Do all febrile infants require hospitalization?

Answer

No, the Boston, Philadelphia, or Rochester criteria can identify infants that are at low risk for serious bacterial illness and provide options for outpatient management.

CHAPTER 48: RISK OF SERIOUS BACTERIAL INFECTION IN FEBRILE INFANTS WITH RSV

Risk of Serious Bacterial Infection in Young Febrile Infants With Respiratory Syncytial Virus Infections

Levine DA, Platt SL, Dayan PS, et al. *Pediatrics.* 2004;113(6):1728–1734

BACKGROUND
Fever can be the only marker of impending septicemia and a key cause of infant mortality. It is challenging to identify neonates at high risk of sepsis from those with more benign etiologies of fever. Although this challenge had been partially addressed by the Rochester, Philadelphia, and Boston criteria, these diagnostic protocols require invasive testing. At the time of this study, it was unclear whether having a diagnosed viral illness, such as Respiratory syncytial virus (RSV), lowered the risk for having a serious bacterial infection (SBI).

OBJECTIVES
To determine the risk of SBI in febrile infants with RSV.

METHODS
Prospective, multicenter, cross-sectional study at eight pediatric EDs in the United States between 1998 and 2001.

Patients
1,248 infants ≤60 days who were found to be febrile with rectal temperature ≥38°C. Select exclusion criteria: Antibiotics within 48 hours prior to enrollment, refusal of consent (missed patients), or RSV or bacterial cultures that were not obtained (failed protocol).

Intervention Evaluated
Patients had nasopharyngeal aspirates screened for RSV, blood cultures, and urinalysis via catheterization and lumbar puncture. Stool cultures and chest radiographs were done at the discretion of the treating physician.

Outcomes
The primary outcome was to determine the risk of SBI in RSV-positive patients. The RSV rates in relation to SBI were analyzed. RSV status was determined by positive rapid immunoassay. SBI was defined as presence of bacterial meningitis, urinary tract infection (UTI), bacteremia, or bacterial enteritis. Pneumonia was not included in the definition of SBI.

KEY RESULTS
- The RSV-positive group ($n = 269$) had a lower rate of SBI when compared to the RSV-negative group (7% vs. 12.5%).
- In RSV-positive patients with SBI, UTI was the most common cause at 5.4%. There were no cases of bacterial meningitis in the RSV-positive group.
- The rate of SBI in infants ≤28 days did not differ significantly between RSV-positive and RSV-negative groups (10.1 vs. 14.2).

STUDY CONCLUSIONS
Febrile infants ≤60 days of age with RSV infections are at lower risk for SBI than those without.

COMMENTARY
Febrile infants continue to present a diagnostic challenge to the emergency physician. Several studies have evaluated viral illnesses' relationship to SBI to help diagnostic efficiency in these patients, but none had applied a prospective, standardized protocol in the ED. This study suggests that febrile infants 28 to 60 days with RSV-positive testing may only need catheterized urine to identify SBI, which dramatically reduces the need for painful lumbar punctures and costly blood and stool cultures. These findings should be interpreted recognizing the limitation that pneumonia was not included in the SBI criteria, and can therefore not guide the decision whether to obtain or forgo chest radiography. In addition, almost 7% of infants with RSV were found to have an SBI which may be too conservative for some physicians. With the understanding that no diagnostic test can completely eliminate the possibility of SBI in a febrile infant, this study helps clinicians efficiently identify children at the highest risk of SBI while reducing potentially harmful or costly testing.

Question
Does a positive RSV test exclude the possibility of a serious bacterial infection in febrile infants?

Answer
No, however, RSV positive infants are significantly less likely to have a SBI. Infants 29 to 60 days of age should undergo a urinalysis. Infants ≤28 days old should undergo a complete evaluation for SBI.

SECTION 7

NEUROLOGY

David Yamane ■ Michael E. Billington

49. CT Before Lumbar Puncture in Meningitis
50. Steroids and Antivirals in Bell's Palsy
51. Prochlorperazine in Migraine
52. Metoclopramide in Migraine
53. tPA for Acute Ischemic Stroke: The NINDS Trial
54. Intra-arterial tPA in Acute Ischemic Stroke: The Proact II Study
55. Timing of tPA in Acute Ischemic Stroke
56. Expanded window for tPA in Stroke: The ECASS III Study
57. Determining Stroke Risk After TIA: The ABCD Score
58. Urgent Follow up for TIA: The EXPRESS Study
59. The Epley Maneuver for Vertigo
60. Risk of Seizure Recurrence in Pediatrics

CHAPTER 49
CT BEFORE LUMBAR PUNCTURE IN MENINGITIS

Computed Tomography of the Head Before Lumbar Puncture in Adults With Suspected Meningitis
Hasbun R, Abrahams J, Jekel J, Quagliarello VJ. *N Engl J Med.* 2001;345(24):1727–1733

BACKGROUND
At the time of this study, CT scan was routinely preformed in patients suspected of having bacterial meningitis prior to performing lumbar puncture (LP). It was thought that this was critical to identifying occult intracranial abnormalities that could put the patient at risk for brain herniation caused by the LP. However, this practice leads to delays in antibiotics and exposes patients to potentially unnecessary cost and radiation. This study sought to determine if there was a subgroup of patients who did not require CT before LP.

OBJECTIVES
To determine if the absence of certain clinical features can identify adults with suspected meningitis who are unlikely to have abnormalities on their CT head.

METHODS
Prospective observational study at a single academic ED in the United States between 1995 and 1999.

Patients
301 patients, >16 years old, with suspected meningitis. Of these, 235 patients underwent CT of the head and 289 underwent LP.

Interventions Evaluated
Structured data collection of clinical features prior to CT of the head.

Outcomes
The primary outcome was a set of clinical features associated with abnormal CT head findings. The secondary outcome was clinical status of the patients at 1 week, including brain herniation.

KEY RESULTS
- The following clinical features were associated with abnormal CT scan of the head:
  - >60 years old
  - Seizure within 1 week of presentation
  - Unable to follow two consecutive commands
  - Facial palsy
  - Immunocompromised (HIV/AIDS, immunosuppressive therapy, transplant)
  - Abnormal level of consciousness
  - Gaze palsy

- Arm drift
- History of CNS disease
- Unable to answer two consecutive questions
- Abnormal visual fields
- Abnormal language
- 40% (96/235) of patients had none of the above findings. Of those, 97% (93/96) had a normal head CT. Of the three patients with abnormal CT scans, two had no mass effect and one had hydrocephalus and mild mass effect.
- Four out of 235 patients had CT findings that caused the clinician to defer an LP, of these two died from herniation despite never undergoing LP.
- Of the 289 patients who underwent LP and had follow-up data available, none had herniation at 1 week. This included seven patients with mild to moderate mass effect on CT head, and all patients who were misclassified based on clinical features.

STUDY CONCLUSIONS

In adults with suspected meningitis, the absence of the specific clinical features can identify patients with low suspicion for abnormal findings on CT head.

COMMENTARY

Historically, the use of CT imaging of the head prior to LP was standard despite limited data to suggest a risk of herniation secondary to procedural effects on intracranial pressures. Beyond prolonging ED evaluations, the routine use of CT prior to LP often delayed the time treating patients with antibiotics. This study identified several features associated with abnormal CT scans to help clinicians safely identify patients in whom CT was not required prior to LP. The strength to this study was that it was prospective, which allowed collection of a wide range of potentially meaningful predictors. These findings have supported the selective use of CT in patients with a high suspicion for bacterial meningitis. The largest limitation to this study is that it was a derivation study and does not have a validation component to it. In addition, the 2004 IDSA guidelines that were developed based on this study also included the absence of papilledema as important to exclude the need for CT—a clinical finding that many emergency physicians feel inadequately trained or resourced to detect in the ED setting. Also, readers should note that the authors designed this study to identify features suggestive of a positive CT scan as a surrogate measure, and not as a study of clinical features in which CT can be excluded or of actual herniation, both of which would have broadened the use of study findings.

Question

Do all patients require CT imaging of the brain prior to lumbar puncture for suspected meningitis?

Answer

No, the absence of select clinical features can identify patients at very low risk for having abnormal CT imaging. It is unclear if abnormal imaging is associated with the risk of herniation.

CHAPTER 50
STEROIDS AND ANTIVIRALS IN BELL'S PALSY

Early Treatment With Prednisolone or Acyclovir in Bell's Palsy
Sullivan F, Swan IR, Donnan P, et al. *N Engl J Med.* 2007;357(16):1598–1607

BACKGROUND
Idiopathic unilateral facial nerve paralysis (Bell's palsy) affects approximately 40,000 Americans per year. Although most patients recover well, as many as 30% are left with a facial disfigurement and ongoing pain. Treatment choices varied and prior to this study, two Cochrane reviews independently concluded that there was insufficient data to support the use of prednisolone, acyclovir, or both in the treatment of Bell's palsy due to lack of evidence.

OBJECTIVES
To determine the efficacy of prednisolone and acyclovir, individually and in combination, in the early treatment of Bell's palsy.

METHODS
Double-blind, placebo-controlled randomized trial conducted across 17 hospitals in Scotland.

Patients
Five hundred and fifty-one patients, >16 years old, presenting with unilateral facial nerve weakness of no identifiable cause and referred to a collaborating ENT within 72 hours from the onset of symptoms. Select exclusion criteria: Pregnancy, breast-feeding, uncontrolled diabetes, herpes zoster, or systemic infection.

Intervention Evaluated
Patients were randomly assigned to receive 10 days of prednisolone; 10 days of acyclovir; 10 days of prednisolone + acyclovir, or placebo.

Outcomes Measured
The primary outcome was recovery of facial function, as measured by the House–Brackmann grading system for facial nerve function. Secondary outcomes were quality of life, appearance, and pain. Outcomes were assessed at 3 and 9 months.

KEY RESULTS
- At 3 months, there was a statistically significant improvement in facial function recovery in patients who received prednisolone compared to those who did not receive prednisolone (83% vs. 63.6%).

- There was no difference in facial function recovery between patients who received acyclovir compared to placebo (71.2% vs. 75.7%; $p = 0.50$).
- At 9 months, the same relationship was seen (prednisolone group, 94.4% vs. no prednisolone, 81.6%; acyclovir group, 85.4% vs. no acyclovir, 90.8%; $p = 0.10$).
- For patients treated with both prednisolone and acyclovir, there was no added benefit of acyclovir compared to prednisolone alone (3 month $p = 0.32$; 9 month $p = 0.72$).
- There were no significant differences among the groups in the secondary outcomes of quality of life, appearance, and pain.

STUDY CONCLUSIONS

When given early in the course of Bell's palsy, prednisolone significantly improves facial function recovery compared to placebo. Acyclovir alone is no different than placebo, and when given in combination with prednisolone, provides no added benefit.

COMMENTARY

Prior to this study, there was widespread variation in and controversy over the treatment of Bell's palsy, and two Cochrane reviews pooling together data from multiple studies deemed that there was insufficient evidence to support the use of either prednisolone or acyclovir. This study was the first to demonstrate clinically important benefits with long-term (9-month) follow-up while utilizing a randomized design. Although there was no difference in quality of life, appearance, or pain between the study groups, this study revealed a significant improvement in facial function with early prednisolone treatment and no added benefit of acyclovir, leading to an American Academy of Neurology Class 1A recommendation for the use of steroids in the treatment of new-onset Bell's palsy.

Question

Is there any effective pharmaceutical intervention for Bell palsy?

Answer

Yes, early treatment with prednisolone significantly improves facial function recovery, while acyclovir does not improve outcomes.

CHAPTER 51
PROCHLORPERAZINE IN MIGRAINE

Randomized, Placebo-Controlled Evaluation of Prochlorperazine vs. Metoclopramide for Emergency Department Treatment of Migraine Headache
Coppola M, Yealy DM, Leibold RA. *Ann Emerg Med.* 1995;26(5):541–546

BACKGROUND
Migraine is a common disease, affecting 29.5 million American adults, and resulting in over $700 million from migraine-related ED visits. Prochlorperazine, an antipsychotic of the phenothiazine class, and metoclopramide, a dopamine antagonist, are both used in the ED treatment of migraine; however, prior to this study it was not known which agent was superior in the treatment of migraine.

OBJECTIVES
To compare prochlorperazine and metoclopramide in the ED treatment of migraine.

METHODS
Prospective randomized double-blind placebo-controlled trial at a single US academic ED.

Patients
Seventy patients, between 18 and 65 years old, presenting with migraine headache similar to prior episodes with or without nausea, vomiting, photophobia, or phonophobia. Select exclusion criteria: Pregnancy, fever, meningismus, altered mental status, use of analgesics, drugs, or alcohol within 24 hours, oxygen saturation <90%, trauma or seizure within 24 hours, and hypertension.

Intervention Evaluated
Patients were randomized to receive 10-mg IV prochlorperazine, 10-mg IV metoclopramide, or saline solution of equal volume. Patients scored their pain, nausea, and sedation on a 0–10 scale prior to the intervention and 30 minutes later. Patients without clinical improvement after 30 minutes were treated at the discretion of the physician.

Outcomes Measured
The primary outcome was clinically relevant and successful treatment, defined as patient satisfaction and either a decrease in pain score by 50% or an absolute pain score after treatment of 2.5 or less.

KEY RESULTS
- Successful treatment occurred most often with prochlorperazine (82%) compared to metoclopramide (48%) or placebo (29%).
- At 30 minutes, median pain scores were significantly less in the prochlorperazine group (prochlorperazine, 1.1; metoclopramide, 3.9; placebo, 6.1).

- At 30 minutes, median nausea scores tended to be less in the prochlorperazine group compared to metoclopramide or placebo ($p = 0.15$).
- At 30 minutes, median sedation scores were not significantly different between the groups ($p = 0.64$).
- Success rates of metoclopramide and placebo were not significantly different ($p = 0.37$).

STUDY CONCLUSIONS

IV prochlorperazine provides better pain relief and tends to alleviate nausea more than IV metoclopramide in the treatment of ED patients with migraine.

COMMENTARY

Prior to this study, there was significant debate in the literature regarding the efficacy of metoclopramide in acute migraine; several studies showed that metoclopramide was more effective than placebo, but much of the data regarding pain or nausea reduction compared to other agents used in acute migraine were either not statistically significant or obtained from very small or flawed studies from which no real conclusions can be made.[1] Although this is a small study, it does show that prochlorperazine provided significantly superior pain relief and increased rates of successful treatment in acute migraine compared to metoclopramide. In fact, success rates of metoclopramide and placebo were not significantly different. This study suggests that the first line of treatment for acute migraine patients in the ED should be prochlorperazine. However, a subsequent paper in the Annals of Emergency Medicine showed noninferiority between 20-mg IV metoclopramide and 10-mg IV prochlorperazine, so the effect described in this study may have been a dosing limitation.[2] Taken in concert with other literature, these findings support current guidelines favoring nonopiate approaches to acute migraine in the ED.

Question

Which treatment is more efficacious for acute migraine in the ED: Prochlorperazine or metoclopramide?

Answer

Prochlorperazine provides better pain relief and tends to alleviate nausea more than metoclopramide; however, this finding may be related to dosing.

References

1. Colman I, Brown MD, Innes GD, Grafstein E, Roberts TE, Rowe BH. Parenteral metoclopramide for acute migraine: Meta-analysis of randomised controlled trials. *BMJ.* 2004;329(7479):1369–1373.
2. Friedman BW, Esses D, Solorzano C, et al. A randomized controlled trial of prochlorperazine versus metoclopramide for treatment of acute migraine. *Ann Emerg Med.* 2008;52(4):399–406.

CHAPTER 52
METOCLOPRAMIDE IN MIGRAINE

Metoclopramide vs. Hydromorphone for the Emergency Department Treatment of Migraine Headache
Griffith J, Mycyk MB, Kyriacou DN. *J Pain.* 2008;9(1):88–94

BACKGROUND
Twenty-eight million Americans suffer from headaches, and of these 15% seek ED evaluation at some point. Migraine headaches account for more than $17 billion in health care costs in the United States annually. At the time of this study, previously used treatments such as prochlorperazine and droperidol were not readily available secondary to shortages and black box warnings. Hydromorphone was often used, however, it was acknowledged that nonopiate options were preferable given the risk of addiction and adverse effects. Metoclopramide was identified as a useful abortive treatment but had not been studied in the ED setting.

OBJECTIVES
To compare the effectiveness of metoclopramide vs. hydromorphone for the initial treatment of migraine in ED patients.

METHODS
Retrospective cohort study at a single academic medical center in the United States.

Participants
200 subjects, 18 to 79 years old, with ICD-9 diagnosis of migraine or who met the diagnostic criteria for migraine by the international classification of headache disorders. Select exclusion criteria: Fever >100.5° F, meningeal signs, altered mental status, focal neurologic deficit, antecedent trauma, pregnancy, or breast-feeding.

Intervention Evaluated
Metoclopramide, hydromorphone, and all other combined medications were compared. Other medications included promethazine, ondansetron, sumatriptan, ibuprofen, ketorolac, hydrocodone/acetaminophen, acetaminophen, prochlorperazine, meperidine, acetaminophen with butalbital and caffeine, and magnesium.

Outcomes
The primary outcome was the difference in selfreported pain scores (on a 0–10 scale) at triage, before medication, at administration, and after medication administration. A reduction of more than 3 was deemed clinically effective. Secondary outcomes included administration of rescue medication, adverse reaction, and time to discharge after administration of initial treatment.

KEY RESULTS
- 26% (51) received hydromorphone (IM or IV), 48% (95) received metoclopramide, and 27% (54) received one or more other medications.
- There was a greater mean reduction in pain scores for metoclopramide (3.7) vs. hydromorphone (2.3) and other medications (2.8).
- Metoclopramide was more clinically effective in treatment of migraines when compared to hydromorphone, with a crude relative risk reduction of 1.76 ($p = 0.01$), and adjusted relative risk of 1.60 ($p = 0.15$).
- Metoclopramide resulted in less use of rescue medications and faster times to discharge. There was no difference in adverse reactions.

STUDY CONCLUSIONS
Metoclopramide is an effective treatment of migraine pain and is more effective than hydromorphone.

COMMENTARY
Prior to this study, metoclopramide was considered inferior to prochlorperazine for acute migraine, however, due to national shortages of prochlorperazine, metoclopramide and hydromorphone had increasing use in the treatment of migraines. This study showed the superiority of metoclopramide over hydromorphone in the treatment of migraines, and provided clinical evidence to support the clinical refrain to avoid opiate therapy in patients with acute migraine. This initial work was retrospective, which does not allow for the standardization of treatment dose, route, and timing; however, subsequent to this work numerous prospective and randomized studies have continued to demonstrate efficacy in the treatment of acute migraine in the ED.

Question
Are dopaminergic agents superior to opiates as a treatment for acute migraine in the ED?

Answer
Yes, in comparison to hydromorphone, metoclopramide leads to a greater reduction in pain scores.

CHAPTER 53
tPA FOR ACUTE ISCHEMIC STROKE: THE NINDS TRIAL

Tissue Plasminogen Activator for Acute Ischemic Stroke.
The National Institute of Neurological Disorders and Stroke rt-PA Stroke Study Group
N Engl J Med. 1995;333(24):1581–1587

BACKGROUND
Ischemic stroke affects over 400,000 people in the United States annually. At the time of this study, there was no direct treatment to reduce neurologic injury. Early trials of thrombolytic therapy showed intracerebral hemorrhage to be a major complication and the magnitude of clinical benefit with respect to mortality was not well-known. However, prior trials suggested that use within 180 minutes was relatively safe and warranted a wider and more rigorous study.

OBJECTIVES
To determine if IV tPA has improved clinical outcome if administered within 3 hours of onset of stroke symptoms.

METHODS
Randomized double-blinded trial conducted in eight centers around the United States between 1991 and 1994. The study was divided into two parts, one to detect an early effect (<24 hours) and the second to detect a late effect (3 months).

Participants
Six hundred and twenty-four patients presenting within 3 hours of stroke symptoms, deficit measurable on the NIH Stroke Scale (NIHSS) and a baseline CT brain without hemorrhage. Two hundred and ninety-one patients were included in part 1 and 333 patients were included in part 2. Select exclusion criteria: Stroke or serious head trauma within 3 months, major surgery, history of intracerebral hemorrhage, SBP >185 mm Hg, DBP >100 mm Hg, rapidly improving or minor symptoms, GI or urinary hemorrhage within 21 days, seizure at onset of stroke, taking anticoagulants, platelets <100,000, or glucose <50 or >400.

Intervention Evaluated
Patients were randomized to receive placebo or recombinant tPA.

Outcomes
Part 1 assessed change in neurologic deficits after 24 hours, indicated by improvement of 4 points on NIHSS. Part 2 assessed sustained clinical benefit after 3 months, using four scales (Barthel Index, modified Rankin scale, Glasgow outcome, and NIHSS).

KEY RESULTS
- Part 1 showed no significant difference in improvement of neurologic deficits at 24 hours between tPA and placebo.
- Part 2 showed favorable neurologic outcome at 90 days with tPA when compared to placebo, with an odds ratio 1.7.
- Symptomatic hemorrhage within 36 hours occurring in 6.4% of tPA patients vs. 0.6% of placebo patients.
- There was no significant difference in mortality at 3 months (17% in the tPA group vs. 21% in the placebo group, $p = 0.30$).

STUDY CONCLUSIONS
In ischemic stroke, IV tPA given within 3 hours of onset of symptoms leads to improved clinical outcome at 3 months despite having an increased incidence of symptomatic intracranial hemorrhage.

COMMENTARY
Unlike myocardial ischemia, for which early use of thrombolysis markedly improved morbidity and mortality, the same was not originally true for cerebral ischemia. This landmark trial was used to support FDA approval and widespread use of tPA for acute ischemic stroke within 3 hours of symptom onset. The initial findings of this trial were interpreted with caution because benefit was only shown in neurologic outcomes at 3 months but not in mortality or 24-hour neurologic outcomes. The lack of mortality difference can largely be attributed to the greater than 6% symptomatic hemorrhage rate for patients treated with tPA, many of which were fatal. Beyond FDA approval, these findings helped spur the development of acute stroke protocols, the formation of stroke center, and national campaigns to improve stroke care.

Question
Does IV tPA improve outcomes in ED patients with acute stroke?

Answer
Yes, IV tPA results in better 90-day neurologic outcomes when given within 3 hours of symptom onset; however, there is no reduction in mortality.

INTRA-ARTERIAL tPA IN ACUTE ISCHEMIC STROKE: THE PROACT II STUDY

Intra-arterial Prourokinase for Acute Ischemic Stroke. The PROACT II Study: A Randomized Controlled Trial

Furlan A, Higashida R, Wechsler L, et al. *JAMA*. 1999;282(21):2003–2011

BACKGROUND

The NINDS trial shows that intravenous tPA is beneficial when given to appropriate patients within 3 hours of stroke onset, but many acute stroke patients are present outside of this window. Prior to this study, PROACT I showed a mild benefit of intra-arterial prourokinase (IA tPA) if given up to 6 hours after stroke onset. It was thought, however, that a higher dose could increase this efficacy and required randomized study.

OBJECTIVES

To evaluate the efficacy of a higher dose of IA tPA than had previously studied in the PROACT I trial, as a therapy for acute middle cerebral artery (MCA) stroke patients who present within 6 hours of symptom onset.

METHODS

Open-label, randomized controlled trial with blinded follow-up conducted at 54 centers in the United States and Canada.

Participants

One hundred and eighty patients 18 to 65 years old with acute ischemic stroke, NIH Stroke Scale (NIHSS) of 4 or greater (except for isolated aphasia or hemianopia), <6 hours of symptoms, and angiographically proven MCA occlusion. Select exclusion criteria: NIHSS >30, coma, rapidly improving neurologic symptoms, history of intracranial hemorrhage, surgery/lumbar puncture within 30 days, head trauma within 90 days, coagulopathy, uncontrolled hypertension, and intracranial tumor/hemorrhage/infarction on CT imaging.

Intervention Evaluated

Patients were randomized to receive either IA tPA via MCA microcatheter and IV heparin or IV heparin alone.

Outcomes Measured

The primary outcome was slight or no neurologic disability at 90 days, as defined by a modified Rankin scale of 2 or less. The secondary outcomes were MCA recanalization, intracranial hemorrhage with neurologic deterioration, and mortality.

KEY RESULTS
- Forty percent of IA tPA patients had a modified Rankin scale of 2 or less, compared to 25% of control patients ($p = 0.04$).
- Recanalization rate was substantially higher in the IA tPA group (66% vs. 18%).
- Mortality was lower in the IA tPA group (25% vs. 27%)
- ICH with neurologic deterioration within 24 hours occurred in more of the IA tPA group (10% vs. 2%); ($p = 0.06$), equating to a number needed to harm of 12.

STUDY CONCLUSIONS
Treatment of IA tPA was beneficial in MCA stroke of less than 6 hours duration despite an increased risk of early intracranial hemorrhage with neurologic deterioration.

COMMENTARY
Given that many patients presents to the ED too late for IV tPA therapy, this study was designed to identify an alternative therapy for acute ischemic stroke patients with severe strokes. In addition to better neurologic outcomes, the intra-arterial group had increased rates of MCA recanalization and similar mortality compared to the control group.

There was an increased rate of early intracranial hemorrhage seen in the intra-arterial group, though the authors note that there was no significant difference between the rates of total intracranial hemorrhage in the intra-arterial and placebo groups by study day 10.

The widespread applications of these findings have been limited by the need for advanced imaging and treatment at specialized centers to use intra-arterial tPA, which are often challenging for patients to arrive at within 6 hours. It is unclear whether these results generalize to ischemic strokes in other vessel territories or for strokes with lower NIHSS but notable disability.

This study led to a change in the American Heart Association/American Stroke Association guidelines for the management of acute stroke to include a class 1B recommendation of intra-arterial thrombolysis for appropriate patients.

Question
Is there an effective intervention for acute stroke patients presenting to the ED outside the traditional 3-hour IV tPA window?

Answer
Yes, patients with an acute middle cerebral artery ischemic stroke who are treated with intra-arterial tPA between 3 and 6 hours of symptom onset demonstrate better 90-day neurologic outcomes.

CHAPTER 55
TIMING OF tPA IN ACUTE ISCHEMIC STROKE

Association of Outcome With Early Stroke Treatment: Pooled Analysis of ATLANTIS, ECASS, and NINDS rt-PA Stroke Trials
Hacke W, Donnan G, Fieschi C, et al. *Lancet.* 2004;363:768–774

BACKGROUND
Ischemic stroke is the one of the leading causes of death in the US, and a disease that has only one acute treatment that has ever been FDA approved. The landmark study (National Institute of Neurological Disorders and Stroke [NINDS]) to establish the efficacy of IV tPA only established benefit for patients treated within 3 hours of stroke onset. Unfortunately few patients reach the ED with enough time for treatment in this time window. At the time of this study, there was conflicting evidence to support treatment with IV tPA for all strokes beyond 3 hours, and no definitive study exploring the relationship between the time to treatment and the efficacy of tPA.

OBJECTIVES
To determine whether the time between symptom onset and treatment with IV tPA is a predictor of therapeutic benefit, and to further clarify the appropriate cut off for tPA treatment.

METHODS
Meta-analysis of six large, multicenter, randomized controlled trials conducted in the United States, Europe, and North America.

Participants
27,775 patients, at >300 hospitals from 18 countries. The data came from the NINDS studies, parts 1 and 2 (3-hour window), ECASS trials, parts 1 and 2 (6-hour window), ATLANTIS trials part A (6-hour window) and B (5-hour window). Varying exclusion criteria based on tPA contraindications (preceding stroke, head trauma, major surgery, history of intracerebral hemorrhage, elevated BP, anticoagulants, thrombocytopenia, anemia).

Intervention Evaluated
All studies (NINDS, ATLANTIS [A and B], ECASS I and II) evaluated varying doses of tPA vs. placebo.

OUTCOMES
The primary outcome was favorable 3-month outcome. Favorable outcome was defined by three neurologic functions scored: Modified Rankin scale (0 or 1), Barthel Index (95 or 100), and NIHSS (0 or 1). The secondary outcomes were intracerebral hemorrhage and death.

KEY RESULTS
- Favorable outcome for tPA compared to controls had the following odds ratios for symptom onset to treatment time:
  - 2.81 for 0 to 90 minutes
  - 1.55 for 91 to 180 minutes
  - 1.4 for 181 to 270 minutes
  - 1.2 for 271 to 360 minutes
- The hazard ratio for death was not significantly different (1) for symptom onset to treatment of 0 to 90 minutes, 91 to 180 minutes, 181 to 270 minutes; however, for 271 to 360 minutes it was 1.45.
- ICH was associated with tPA treatment (vs. placebo) and age but not associated with time to treatment.

STUDY CONCLUSIONS
There is a relation between symptom onset to treatment time and favorable neurologic outcome, and early treatment with tPA is associated with more favorable outcomes. This also implies that there is neurologic benefit to treatment of acute ischemic stroke beyond 3 hours.

COMMENTARY
While rt-tPA had shown some efficacy and gained FDA approval for patients with acute ischemic stroke presenting within 3 hours of symptom, there was marked resistance to widespread use because many clinicians were suspicious of the benefits of treatment given high rates of ICH and because many patients present to the ED too late for therapy. This meta-analysis confirmed earlier findings of treatment benefit within 3 hours of symptom onset in a pooled, more generalizable population. In addition, the six trials pooled in this analysis enabled assessment of multiple treatment windows that shows the potential for favorable neurologic outcomes in patients treated outside the 3-hour window. This study was influential to promote further studies to expand rt-tPA use beyond the 3-hour window for ischemic stroke.

Question
What is the optimal treatment window for tPA in acute ischemic stroke?

Answer
Consistent with the original NINDS study, favorable neurologic outcomes are associated with treatment within 4.5 hours of symptom onset and greater efficacy if treated within 3 hours.

CHAPTER 56
EXPANDED WINDOW FOR tPA IN STROKE: THE ECASS III STUDY

Thrombolysis With Alteplase 3 to 4.5 Hours After Acute Ischemic Stroke
Hacke W, Kaste M, Bluhmki E, et al. *N Engl K Med.* 2008;359(13):1317–1329

BACKGROUND
In 1995 the NINDS trial showed that patients treated with Alteplase (tPA) within 3 hours of onset of stroke symptoms were 30% more likely to have minimal or no disability at 3 months. International guidelines recommend tPA as first-line treatment for all eligible patients; however, fewer than 2% patients received this intervention, mostly due to delay in presentation to a stroke center. Extending the treatment window became a goal for subsequent research. The ECASS and ECASS II trials investigated the use of tPA up to 6 hours but failed to show efficacy. Some small randomized trials and the pooled analysis in the prior study showed favorable outcomes between 3 and 4.5 hours but clarification of the timing and patient population was needed.

OBJECTIVES
To test the efficacy and safety of tPA between 3 and 4.5 hours after the onset of stroke symptoms.

METHODS
Double-blind, parallel group trial, from 130 centers across 19 European countries.

Participants
Eight hundred and twenty-one patients, 18 to 80 years old, with the clinical diagnosis of acute ischemic stroke between 3 and 4.5 hours. Four hundred and eighteen patients received tPA and 403 received placebo. Select exclusion criteria: Intracranial hemorrhage (ICH) or major ischemic infarction (NIHSS >25).

Interventions Evaluated
Patients were randomly assigned to receive IV tPA or placebo between 3 and 4.5 hours of symptom onset of ischemic stroke.

Outcomes
The primary outcome was disability at 90 days measured on the modified Rankin scale (0 or 1 meaning no or little disability). Secondary outcomes included combined outcomes at 90 days measured on the Barthel index, NIHSS, and Glasgow outcome scale. Safety outcomes were overall mortality, any ICH, symptomatic ICH, and symptomatic edema.

KEY RESULTS
- More patients in the tPA group had little or no disability at 90 days when compared with placebo (52.4% vs. 44.2%).
- The tPA group had a higher incidence of both ICH (27% vs. 17.6%) and symptomatic ICH (2.4% vs. 0.2%) when compared to placebo.
- There was no difference in mortality between the two groups (7.7% in the tPA group vs. 8.4% in placebo group; $p = 0.68$).

STUDY CONCLUSIONS
IV tPA is effective in the treatment of acute ischemic stroke when given from 3 to 4.5 hours. Despite a higher incidence of ICH and symptomatic ICH in the tPA group, it was no higher than previous studies suggested and there was no difference in mortality between the groups.

COMMENTARY
Prior to this study, the use of tPA in ischemic stroke was limited to a time window of 3 hours since onset of symptoms based on the original NINDS trial. As stroke care improved through the organization of stroke care systems, observational research utilizing advanced MRI imaging had demonstrated that many patients continued to be at risk of ischemia beyond the 3-hour window, creating an impetus for this study to evaluate broader use of tPA therapy. This study was a well-designed and executed randomized trial supporting extension of the tPA treatment window to 4.5 hours for select patients (patients with diabetes, history of previous stroke, or those with severe stroke). Clinicians should also note that the risk of ICH was considerably higher, however, very few were symptomatic, in comparison to the ICH rates reported in studies of patients treated within the 3-hour window. Given that the majority of patients had little or no disability at 90 days, these findings have supported wider use of tPA within 4.5 hours for select patients treated at stroke centers.

Question
Can the use of IV tPA in the treatment of acute ischemic stroke be extended from a 3-hour window to a 4.5-hour window?

Answer
Yes, in select patients under age 80 suffering a mild stroke the use of IV tPA between 3 and 4.5 hours after symptom onset can improve 90-day neurologic outcomes.

DETERMINING STROKE RISK AFTER TIA: THE ABCD SCORE

CHAPTER 57

Validation of the ABCD Score in Identifying Individuals at High Early Risk of Stroke After a Transient Ischemic Attack: A Hospital-based Case Series Study
Tsivigoulis G, Spengos K, Manta P, et al. *Stroke.* 2006;37:2892–2897

BACKGROUND
Stroke is a major cause of mortality, and transient ischemic attach (TIA) can be a warning sign of future stroke. A number of possible clinical predictors of stroke risk in patients with a TIA were obtained from the 1991 Oxfordshire Community Stroke Project and led to the development of the ABCD score. This score took clinic-recorded TIA presenting signs and correlated them with subsequent occurrence of stroke. At the time of this study, it was still unknown if this score could be applied to an acute hospital setting and whether it could be used to rule out low-risk patients.

OBJECTIVES
To discriminate between patients who have a high risk of stroke after presenting with a TIA and require emergent work up from those who can be managed with outpatient follow-up.

METHODS
Retrospective blinded single center study of patients presenting to the ED of a neurology department at the University of Athens, Greece, between 2000 and 2004.

Participants
Two hundred and twenty-six consecutive patients who presented to the ED who met WHO definition of TIA.

Intervention Evaluated
Two authors blinded to the outcomes of patients reviewed ED and hospital records of all 226 patients and applied the ABCD score to each chart.
  ABCD Stroke Risk Score (0 to 6 points) Table 57.1
- A: Age: 60 (1)
- B: Blood pressure: BP >140/90 (1)
- C: Clinical: Unilateral weakness (2); speech disturbance without weakness (1); other (0)
- D: Duration: 1 hour (2); 10 to 59 minutes (1); <10 minutes (0)

Outcomes
Diagnosis of stroke at 30 days was defined at symptoms lasting >24 hours with brain imaging confirming a new lesion in an anatomic site or vascular territory unaffected on initial admission CT scan. Secondary outcomes included length of hospital stay, use of prior medications, and known additional stroke risk factors (diabetes, hyperlipidemia).

KEY RESULTS
- Eight percent (18/226) of all patients had strokes within 7 days of TIA; 10% (22/226) had strokes within 30 days.
- No patients with ABCD scores of 2 or less had strokes at 7 or 10 days.
- ABCD score of 5 to 6 conferred a hazard ratio of 8.01 compared to an ABCD score of 0 to 4.
- Removal of the patients with CT changes after TIA ($n = 3$) did not attenuate the predictive value of the ABCD score.
- Presence of diabetes mellitus conferred at hazard ratio of 2.98; hyperlipidemia conferred a hazard ratio 3.83.

STUDY CONCLUSIONS
A high ABCD score (5 to 6) is predictive of a high risk of 7- and 30-day stroke; a low ABCD score (1 to 2) confers a very low risk of stroke at 7 and 30 days. Diabetes and hyperlipidemia were also independent risk factors for stroke.

COMMENTARY
This study was designed to externally validate a stroke risk stratification tool, as well as to identify patients safe for outpatient evaluation and follow-up. The ABCD score was analytically developed from a large database of stroke data collected from the Oxfordshire Community Stroke Project in the 1980s. This project drew from a database of over 100,000 patients and 50 primary care providers across a multiyear survey. The authors of this paper note that their in-hospital stroke incidence as well as 30-day stroke risk compare well to the population studied in Oxfordshire supporting the generalizability of this and earlier work. This study was critical in establishing the ABCD score as a routine screening metric in all patients with ED presentations concerning for TIA. In addition, this study found that diabetes was an independent risk factor for stroke after TIA, and this was incorporated into the subsequently developed, more sensitive ABCD2 score. In addition to providing meaningful risk stratification, use of the ABCD score has been facilitated by its simple construction that does not require specialized laboratory or radiographic equipment for application. As routine neuroimaging becomes more common and available, it is likely that future risk stratification tools will incorporate these and other emerging biomarkers into clinical practice.

Question
Can the clinical characteristics of patients with TIAs be used to identify those at high risk of stroke?

Answer
Yes, the ABCD score provides a simple, clinically based tool that can risk stratify and differentiate between patients requiring inpatient hospitalization and outpatient management.

Table 57.1 ABCD2 Scoring Criteria

A Age	≥60 yr	1 point
B Blood pressure	≥140/90 mm Hg	1 point
C Clinical features	Unilateral weakness	2 points
	Speech impairment without weakness	1 point
D Duration	≥60 min	2 points
	10–59 min	1 point
D Diabetes	Presence of diabetes mellitus	1 point

Low risk (0 to 3 points), medium risk (4 to 5 points), and high risk (6 to 7 points)

CHAPTER 58
URGENT FOLLOW UP FOR TIA: THE EXPRESS STUDY

Effect of Urgent Treatment of Transient Ischaemic Attack and Minor Stroke on Early Recurrent Stroke (EXPRESS Study): A Prospective Population-based Sequential Comparison

Rothwell PM, Giles MF, Chandratheva A, et al. *Lancet.* 2007;370(9596):1432–1442

BACKGROUND
The risk of recurrent stroke in the week after transient ischemic attack (TIA) is up to 10%. Multiple treatments are known to prevent stroke after TIA, including aspirin, antihypertensives, statins, anticoagulation for atrial fibrillation, and carotid endarterectomy. The ABCD study provided emergency clinicians with a risk stratification tool for stroke at 7 and 30 days, but there was a high degree of variation in the urgency with which preventive therapies were initiated after TIA. This varied from emergent inpatient management to routine nonurgent outpatient care. This study sought to quantify the suspected benefits of rapid treatment.

OBJECTIVES
To assess the effect of rapid treatment after TIA.

METHODS
Prospective observational study nested within OXVASC, a longitudinal, population-based observational study of TIA and stroke among nine primary care practices in Oxfordshire, UK.

Participants
1,278 patients referred by primary care physicians to the TIA/stroke clinic due to suspected TIA who did not require inpatient admission.

Intervention Evaluated
In phase 1, patients were referred to a by-appointment-only TIA/stroke clinic that made treatment recommendations to each patient's primary care physician. In phase 2, patients were referred directly to the TIA/stroke clinic without an appointment, and treatment was initiated, including aspirin, simvastatin, antihypertensives, and anticoagulation if indicated, in the clinic if TIA/minor stroke was confirmed.

Outcomes Measured
The risk of stroke within 90 days of first presentation.

KEY RESULTS
- Median delay to assessment in TIA/stroke clinic was less in the rapid treatment group (less than 1 day vs. 3 days in the nonurgent group).
- Median delay to first treatment prescription was less in the rapid treatment group (1 day vs. 20 days in the nonurgent group).
- 90-day risk of recurrent stroke was less in the rapid treatment group (2.1% vs. 10.3% in the nonurgent group).
- Early treatment did not increase the risk of intracerebral hemorrhage.

STUDY CONCLUSIONS
Early treatment after TIA or minor stroke is associated with an 80% reduction in early recurrent stroke.

COMMENTARY
Despite knowledge that the risk of early recurrent stroke is high following a TIA or minor stroke, the impact of early therapy was previously unknown and the value of secondary prevention was unclear. This study changed the emergency management of TIA/minor stroke, highlighting the need for urgent specialist or primary care provider follow-up and early initiation of indicated treatment. These findings may not be wholly generalizable to the ED as patients were enrolled in the ambulatory primary care setting in which diagnostic and risk stratification tools available in the ED are not used, but the strict enrollment criteria suggest that these patients with TIA are very similar. As patients with TIAs and suspected stroke increasingly seek care in the ED, their study demonstrates the importance for emergency care providers to establish protocols and care delivery pathways for patients to ensure timely follow-up and early secondary prevention treatment to reduce stroke recurrence.

Question
Does early follow-up improve long-term outcomes for patients with a TIA or acute stroke?

Answer
Yes, early initiation of simple treatments including aspirin, antilipids, and antihypertensive agents can decrease the 90-day risk of stroke.

THE EPLEY MANEUVER FOR VERTIGO

A Randomized Clinical Trial to Assess the Efficacy of the Epley Maneuver in the Treatment of Acute Benign Positional Vertigo
Chang AK, Schoeman G, Hill M. *Acad Emerg Med.* 2004;11(9):918–924

BACKGROUND
Dizziness is a common ED presenting complaint, and the treatment of dizziness in the United States is estimated to cost over $4 billion per year. Benign positional vertigo (BPV) is the most common cause of vertigo. The Epley maneuver was first developed in 1992 and had previously been shown to be a safe and effective treatment for benign position vertigo (BPV) in neurology clinics, but had not been studied in ED patients and was not used in common practice in the ED. This study sought to show whether this simple, low-cost intervention could benefit ED patients who would otherwise need to wait weeks for an appointment in a neurology clinic.

OBJECTIVES
To determine whether the Epley maneuver is an effective treatment for BPV in ED.

METHODS
Prospective, randomized, single-blind placebo-controlled trial at a single US center.

Participants
Twenty-two patients who were >18 years old, had a history consistent with BPV, and had a Hallpike test with either nystagmus or reproduction of vertiginous symptoms. Select exclusion criteria: History suggestive of labyrinthitis or vestibular neuritis (constant for days, nonpositional, follows a viral prodrome, affects hearing in the case of labyrinthitis), evidence of CNS disease, high-grade carotid stenosis, severe neck disease, and restricted mobility.

Intervention Evaluated
Patients were randomized to the Epley maneuver or to a placebo maneuver. Patients in the placebo group with persistent symptoms underwent a rescue Epley maneuver. Before and after interventions, patients were asked to score the severity of their symptoms on a novel 0 to 10 point scale.

Outcomes Measured
The primary outcome was the difference between severity scores between the two groups. The secondary outcome was the improvement in severity score for placebo-group patients after undergoing a rescue Epley maneuver.

KEY RESULTS
- The Epley group had a larger median decrease in vertigo severity score following the maneuver (6 vs. 1).
- Six out of 11 placebo-group patients received a rescue Epley maneuver, with a statistically significant decrease in their severity score following the rescue Epley maneuver ($p = 0.027$).

STUDY CONCLUSIONS
The Epley maneuver is more efficacious than placebo in ED patients with BPV.

COMMENTARY
Despite its long-time use in the ambulatory setting, this study was the first to demonstrate the effectiveness of the Epley maneuver for the treatment of benign positional vertigo (BPPV) in the ED. Benign positional veritgo is a potentially debilitating condition that often requires costly treatment including IV medications, despite little evidence to support benefit for such treatment. The Epley maneuver is safe, low cost, and easily reproduced making its use in the ED attractive. Clinicians have variably adopted these findings due to limited training and experience in performing the procedure and ED workflows that often favor the use of IV medications because they require less time of the busy providers at the bedside. As pressures continue to reduce the costs of acute care, clinicians including nurses and midlevel providers will likely be supported to perform the Epley maneuver in ED patients with vertigo in conjunction with emergency physician-directed evaluation.

Question
Is the Epley maneuver an effective treatment for ED patients with benign positional vertigo?

Answer
Yes, the Epley maneuver is a safe and noninvasive intervention that improves symptoms of vertigo.

CHAPTER 60
RISK OF SEIZURE RECURRENCE IN PEDIATRICS

The Risk of Seizure Recurrence After a First Unprovoked Afebrile Seizure in Childhood: An Extended Follow-up
Shinnar S, Berg AT, Moshe SL, et al. *Pediatrics.* 1996;98:216–225

BACKGROUND
Prior to 1996, reported risk of recurrent seizure after first unprovoked seizure in childhood varied dramatically. This made prognostication difficult and resulted in significant anxiety in parents. At the time of this study, the significance of first unprovoked seizure in childhood was unknown, prompting a search to find better ways of risk-stratifying children.

OBJECTIVES
To assess the risk of recurrent seizure after a first unprovoked seizure in two populations of children: Children with underlying precipitant neurologic stress, and children who would not otherwise be expected to have a seizure.

METHODS
Prospective observational study at five hospitals in several private practice locations in New York City between 1983 and 1992.

Participants
Four hundred and seven children, 1 month to 19 years old, presenting after first unprovoked seizure (no head trauma, no fever). Children with prior provoked seizures (fever, neonatal, febrile) were included. Select exclusion criteria: Children presenting specifically with absence seizures, myoclonic seizures, or infantile spasms.

Intervention
Correlation of characteristics surrounding first seizure were performed for two distinct populations: (1) the remote symptomatic group: Children with static encephalopathy from birth and/or prior neurologic insult (depressed skull fracture, prior stroke, prior ICH) and (2) the crypogenic group: Children with no prior history of neurologic insult/embarrassment. Clinical characteristics evaluated were prior family history of seizure, age of onset, abnormal EEG, onset during sleep, specific symptomatology (Todd paralysis, presentation in status epilepticus) with recurrence of seizure.

Outcomes
Outcome was seizure recurrence (recurrent seizure >24 hours from first) at 2, 5, and up to 8 years from initial event.

KEY RESULTS
- Overall recurrence by 1992: 42% (171/407); median time 5.7 months; 88% occurred within 2 years.
- Risk of recurrence was 68% in the remote symptomatic group vs. 37% in the cryptogenic group.
- High-risk remote symptomatic correlations: History of prior febrile seizures, age <3.
- High-risk cryptogenic correlations: Abnormal EEG, family history, seizure occurring in sleep, age >3.
- Type or duration of seizure, status epilepticus, and time of day was not predictive in either group.

STUDY CONCLUSIONS
In healthy children without underlying neurologic insult, an abnormal EEG (especially in the context of a family history of seizure), a seizure onset during sleep, and age >3 increased the likelihood of recurrence significantly. In children with prior neurologic insult, a history of febrile seizures and age <3 were associated with increased likelihood of recurrence.

COMMENTARY
Prior to this study there was significant conjecture based on case series and clinical experience, but little population-level data with longitudinal follow-up around risks of seizure recurrence in children. This study utilized its large sample size and long-term follow-up to provide meaningful estimates of seizure recurrence to parents seeking guidance amidst the anxiety of a child's first seizure. Importantly, this study occurred prior to the routine initiation of AEDs in children, likely providing a more accurate natural history of the disease(s). In the more common cryptogenic cohort, the data identifies a particularly low-risk subgroup of recurrence: Children with a normal EEG and a seizure occurring while awake. In the remote symptomatic group, a group which already has higher risk for recurrence, clear exacerbating factors of prior history of febrile seizures and age <3 are demonstrated. While this work helps clinicians provide meaningful prognostic information to families, this study does not address whether AED therapy should be initiated in select patients following a first-time seizure.

Question
What factors predict the development of epilepsy in a child presenting after a first-time seizure and without any previous neurologic injury or disease?

Answer
A seizure occurring during sleep, age >3 years, a family history of seizures, or an abnormal EEG all increase the likelihood of future epilepsy.

SECTION 8: OPERATIONS

Christina Wilson ■ Ije Akunyili

61. Chest Pain Protocols in the ED
62. Stress Testing in the ED
63. Social Interventions for Alcohol Abuse

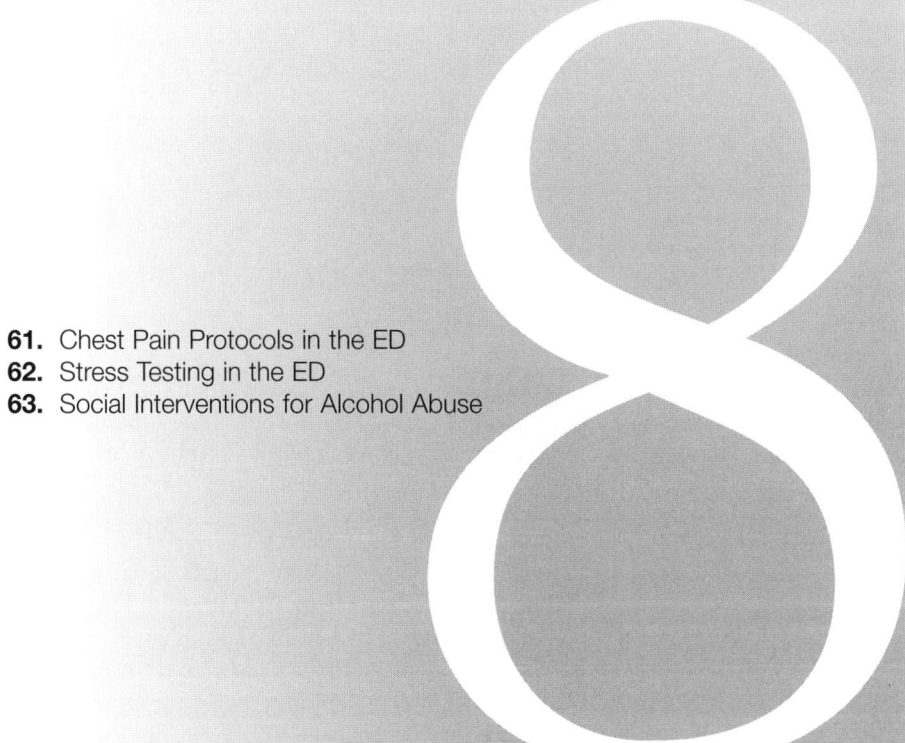

CHAPTER 61
CHEST PAIN PROTOCOLS IN THE ED

Costs of an Emergency Department-based Accelerated Diagnostic Protocol vs. Hospitalization in Patients with Chest Pain
Roberts RR, Zalenski RJ, Mensah EK, et al. *JAMA.* 1997;278(20):1670–1676

BACKGROUND
In the 1990s the majority of patients presenting to the ED with chest pain were hospitalized for further diagnostic testing and risk stratification, with an estimated three million hospitalizations and an annual cost of over three billion dollars for patients ultimately found to be disease free. Previous studies suggested the utility of new cardiac biomarkers and stress testing in the ED had value in evaluating patients with suspected acute myocardial infarction (AMI), but these tools had not been evaluated in a randomized trial. This study developed and tested an accelerated ED diagnostic protocol using these tools.

OBJECTIVES
To determine if the use of an accelerated ED protocol for low-risk patients presenting with chest pain results in reduced hospital admission, cost, and length of stay (LOS) when compared to traditional hospitalization.

METHODS
Prospective, randomized, controlled trial at a large urban public teaching hospital from 1993 to 1995.

Participants
One hundred and sixty-five adult patients presenting to the ED with a presentation suggestive of AMI or acute cardiac ischemia (ACI) who would have otherwise been hospitalized for evaluation per the primary ED attending, with low probability of AMI using the Goldman algorithm, and able to perform an exercise stress test (ETT).

Intervention Evaluated
For the accelerated diagnostic protocol, patients remained in the ED observation unit and had 12 hours of telemetry, CK-MB levels every 4 hours, EKGs and clinical examination every 6 hours, and an ETT. This was compared to standard inpatient care that was 24 hours of telemetry, three sets of cardiac enzymes, two EKGs, and stress testing.

Outcomes
Primary outcomes were LOS and total cost of treatment. Secondary outcomes were hospital admission rate and death within 24 hours.

KEY RESULTS
- The mean total cost per patient for accelerated protocol vs. control patients was $1,528 vs. $2,095.
- The mean LOS for accelerated protocol vs. control patients was 33.1 vs. 44.8 hours.
- The hospital admission rate for accelerated protocol vs. control patients was 45.2% vs. 100%.
- For the subgroup of accelerated protocol patients who were discharged (59%), LOS was 15.7 hours and cost was $803.
- There were no deaths within 24 hours.

STUDY CONCLUSIONS
The use of an accelerated diagnostic protocol in the ED reduces hospitalizations, total LOS, and total costs for low-risk patients with chest pain.

COMMENTARY
This study was practice-changing, providing evidence supporting ED observation protocols for accelerated work-up of presentations otherwise requiring expensive and time-consuming hospitalization. These early accelerated protocols paved the way for the development of chest pain centers and of observation units treating a wide variety of conditions. The accelerated protocol used in this study was conservative when compared to many current chest pain observation unit protocols (with 12 hours of observation, four sets of enzymes, and a stress test), yet still showed a significant improvement in LOS and cost. This effect was amplified for the patients that were safe for discharge. One limitation is that the only secondary outcome studied was death within 24 hours, with no mention of AMI or death at a more distant time period.

Question
Can patients presenting to the ED with acute chest pain be safely evaluated and discharged without inpatient hospitalization?

Answer
Yes, use of an accelerated diagnostic protocol including telemetry, cardiac biomarkers, serial EKGs, and provocative testing is safe and shown to significantly reduce costs and hospital length of stay.

STRESS TESTING IN THE ED

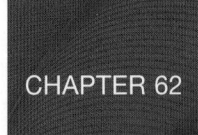

Immediate Exercise Testing of Low Risk Patients with Known Coronary Artery Disease Presenting to the Emergency Department with Chest Pain
Lewis WR, Amsterdam EA, Turnipseed S, Kirk JD. *J Am Coll Cardiol.* 1999;33:1843–1847

BACKGROUND
At the time of this study nearly 3 million patients were admitted in the United States annually for chest pain. Seventy percent of these patients ultimately had a negative cardiac workup. Prior to this study the authors had demonstrated the safety of immediate exercise treadmill testing (ETT) in low-risk patients with no known coronary artery disease (CAD), but it was not yet known if immediate ETT was safe and effective for those with known CAD.

OBJECTIVES
To demonstrate the use and safety of ETT in low-risk patients with known CAD presenting to the ED with chest pain.

METHODS
Prospective observational cohort study conducted in a single US ED from 1993 to 1998.

Patients
One hundred patients with known CAD presenting to the ED with chest pain. Inclusion criteria: Low-risk patients based on initial EKG, clinical findings, and the ability to exercise. Select exclusion criteria: EKG diagnostic of acute myocardial infarction (AMI) or ischemia, EKG with changes that would preclude accurate interpretation of the exercise EKG, and heart failure.

Intervention Evaluated
ETT using 12-lead EKG monitoring and a modified Bruce protocol performed as soon as possible after the emergency physician completed their evaluation. All patients were evaluated with physical examination, chest x-ray, and EKG and most had an initial CK-MB checked.

Outcomes
The primary outcomes were ETT results and rate of AMI. Secondary outcomes included adverse events, rate of admission, and death.

KEY RESULTS
- ETT was positive in 23% (23/100) of patients, nondiagnostic in 39% (39/100), and negative in 38% (38/100).
- No patients with a negative or nondiagnostic ETT were diagnosed with AMI.
- There were no complications from exercise testing.
- 64% (64/100) were discharged immediately after stress testing and 19% (19/100) were discharged in less than 24 hours.
- There were no deaths or AMIs at 6-month follow-up.

STUDY CONCLUSIONS
Select, low-risk patients with known CAD who present to the ED with chest pain can safely undergo ETT for immediate risk stratification.

COMMENTARY
Prior to the advent of ED observation, the standard of care for chest pain was to admit all patients with suspicion of having an AMI to a coronary care unit, with fewer than one-third of these ultimately diagnosed with AMI, at a cost of over 10 billion dollars a year. This study and others provided evidence to pave the way for testing and disposition of patients from the ED that would have otherwise required a full hospital admission. In this study, 64% of patients were able to be discharged immediately after stress testing and none had adverse events, AMI, or death at 6-month follow-up. Of note, all patients in this study had known CAD, which may represent a population at higher risk of AMI than many of the patients currently evaluated in ED chest pain pathways. The high rate of indeterminate stress tests (n = 39) requires mention as well since 17 of these patients required additional observation or admission for cardiac imaging, but none were diagnosed with AMI. In addition to demonstrating the safety of evaluation for AMI in the ED, this study helped set the foundation for a decade of collaboration between emergency physician and cardiologists seeking to develop efficient pathways for the use of cardiac biomarkers, more advanced imaging technologies, and dedicated observation units.

Question
Can immediate stress testing be used in patients with chest pain and known CAD for risk stratification?

Answer
Yes, immediate exercise treadmill testing is safe when applied to the specific population of low-risk patients with known CAD.

CHAPTER 63
SOCIAL INTERVENTIONS FOR ALCOHOL ABUSE

A Brief Intervention Reduces Hazardous and Harmful Drinking in Emergency Department Patients
D'Onofrio G, Fiellin DA, Pantalon MV, et al. *Ann Emerg Med.* 2012;60(2):181–192

BACKGROUND
Brief interventions (BI) are a strategy using existing staff to leverage the authority of medical care providers in helping to change harmful behaviors. One population for whom this shows promise are hazardous and harmful drinkers (HH), an important population to target given that 11,000 (one-third) of the road fatalities in the US are tied to alcohol-impaired driving. The American College of Surgeons requires BIs for all injured patients in level 1 trauma centers. While these strategies have been shown to have efficacy in primary care and trauma inpatient settings, at the time of this study, there had only been small studies with varying methodologies assessing these interventions in the ED. This made them difficult to apply and of uncertain value in a busy ED setting.

OBJECTIVES
To determine the impact of a particular type of BI, the brief negotiation interview (BNI) and a BNI with 1-month follow-up (BNI with booster) on 7-day alcohol consumption and binge-drinking episodes within 28 days.

METHODS
Randomized clinical trial in a US urban teaching hospital.

Patients
Eight hundred and eighty-nine HH drinkers, >18 years old, were randomized. Select exclusion criteria: Patients already enrolled in alcohol treatment, with a life-threatening disorder, suicidal or psychotic, did not speak English, or had alcohol dependence as evidenced by an Alcohol Use Disorders Identification Test (AUDIT) score greater than 19.

Intervention Evaluated
Patients were randomized to the BNI group (n = 297), BNI with booster (n = 295), standard care (SC) (n = 148). A nonassessed standard care (SC-NA) (n = 149) group was also formed to compare to the SC group and control for the impact of assessment.

Outcomes
The primary outcomes were 7-day alcohol consumption and the number of binge-drinking episodes in 28 days. Binge drinking was defined as greater than four drinks per occasion for men and greater than three drinks per occasion for women.

KEY RESULTS
- The BNI with booster had the greatest reduction in mean number of drinks at 7 days, 6 months, and 12 months, followed by the BNI and then SC. The least reduction was seen in the SC-NA group.
  - BNI with booster: 20.4 to 11.6 to 13
  - BNI: 19.8 to 12.7 to 14.3
  - SC: 20.9 to 14.2 to 17.6
- Similarly, reduction in 28-day binge episode was greatest in BNI with booster and BNI group.
- There was no statistically significant difference between the BNI with booster and BNI.
- There was no statistically significant difference between the SC and SC-NA group.

STUDY CONCLUSIONS
BIs performed by the emergency provider can reduce alcohol consumption among HH drinkers.

COMMENTARY
This study was done to prove that even BIs performed in the ED could have a significant impact on the population of HH. The unique contribution of this study is that it adopted a paradigm that was successful in the outpatient setting and applied it to an ED population in a randomized fashion. Papers like this make it imperative that emergency providers be proactive in counseling this subgroup of patients during their time in the ED. Estimating the impact of such intervention studies should always be tempered by the possibility that unblinded providers and investigators may have worked harder to achieve reductions in drinking; however, that would further support the real-world effectiveness of this intervention. While there was an upward trend in drinking habits after several months, this does not negate the importance of BI in the ED. This work demonstrates the importance of the ED at a setting for public health improvement efforts and the opportunity to extend BIs to numerous substance use and behavioral health populations.

Question
Can emergency care providers decrease future alcohol use and improve outcomes in hazardous and harmful drinkers?

Answer
Yes, a brief intervention in the ED even without a follow-up phone call can reduce long-term alcohol use.

SECTION 9
ORTHOPEDICS

Andrew J. Eyre

64. The Ottawa Knee Rules
65. The Ottawa Ankle Rules

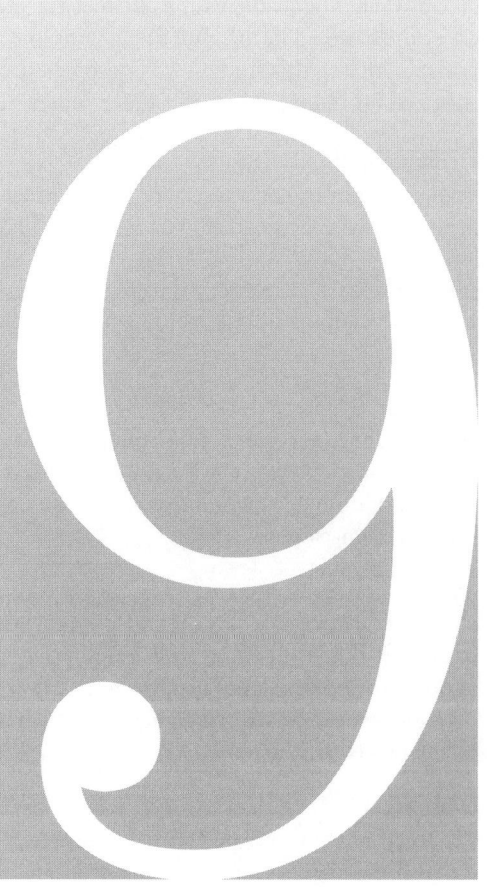

CHAPTER 64 THE OTTAWA KNEE RULES

Derivation of a Decision Rule for the Use of Radiography in Acute Knee Injuries
Stiell IG, Greenberg GH, Wells GA, et al. *Ann Emerg Med.* 1995;26(4):405–413

BACKGROUND
Patients frequently present to the ED with acute knee pain following blunt traumatic injuries and often receive radiographs of the knee as part of their evaluation. The overall fracture rate in these types of injuries is extremely low. One study demonstrated that 94% of knee radiographs in 1,296 patients with knee injuries did not show a fracture. In an era where financial pressures to lower health care costs have become significant drivers of the national health care discussions, the need to introduce selectivity in imaging is critical. Prior to this study, a well-accepted decision rule did not exist to help determine the need for radiography of the knee following blunt knee injuries.

OBJECTIVE
To derive a clinical decision rule to assist in selective radiography of the knee for patients presenting with acute knee pain following blunt injuries.

METHODS
Prospective, observational study conducted in two Canadian EDs between 1992 and 1993.

Patients
A convenience sample of 1,047 adult patients presenting with acute knee injuries from blunt trauma. Select exclusion criteria: Patients with prior imaging, distracting injuries, isolated skin involvement, or patients who had sustained the injuries more than 7 days prior to evaluation.

Intervention Evaluated
Patients were evaluated by attending emergency physicians and assessed for 23 separate criteria. Patients receiving radiography had standard knee X-Rays evaluated by staff radiologists looking for clinically significant fractures. Patients who did not receive radiography were followed with a structured phone interview to determine the possibility of any missed fractures.

Outcomes
Statistical analysis was performed to determine which criteria were most strongly associated with a significant fracture in order to derive the clinical decision rule.

KEY RESULTS
- Five clinical criteria were identified as having the highest association with fracture. These resulted in the development of the Ottawa Knee Rules:

  A knee radiograph is required only for acute knee injury patients with one or more of the following findings:
  - Age 55 years or older
  - Tenderness at the head of the fibula
  - Isolated tenderness of the patella
  - Inability to flex to 90 degrees
  - Inability to bear weight for four steps both immediately and in the ED
- The derived clinical decision rule was 100% sensitive and 54% specific.
- The derived clinical decision rule predicts a 28% reduction in radiography.

STUDY CONCLUSIONS
The Ottawa Ankle Rules identified significant fractures of the knee with 100% sensitivity and 54% specificity in patients presenting with acute knee injuries from blunt trauma.

COMMENTARY
This study introduced a clinical decision rule that could be used to reliably identify patients presenting with acute knee pain from blunt trauma who did not require radiographs as part of their ED evaluation. The Ottawa Knee Rules have since been prospectively validated in a variety of populations and have been integrated into emergency medicine training and practice. While the rules boast 100% sensitivity, the overall utility in daily practice remains unclear. The age criteria (>18 years old) excludes a large number of patients and many patients presenting with acute knee injuries have difficulty localizing tenderness on examination, are reluctant to weight bearing, and have an expectation of receiving radiographs. As clinicians are encouraged to be better stewards of scarce health care resources, the use of clinical guidelines such as the Ottawa Knee and Ankle Rules will take on a more prominent role.

Question
Do all patients who present to the ED with acute knee pain from blunt trauma require radiography to rule out a fracture?

Answer
No, the Ottawa Knee Rules can identify patients at low risk for significant fracture, obviating the need for imaging.

CHAPTER 65: THE OTTAWA ANKLE RULES

Decision Rules for the Use of Radiography in Acute Ankle Injuries. Refinement and Prospective Validation
Stiell IG, Greenberg GH, McKnight RD, et al. *JAMA*. 1993;269(9):1127–1132

BACKGROUND
Ankle injuries are a common presenting complaint in the ED and radiographs of the ankle are among the most commonly ordered radiographic studies. However, the overall fracture rate is less than 15%. Prior to this study, an accepted and validated clinical decision rule did not exist to help determine which patients were at a high risk of fracture, and should receive radiographs.

OBJECTIVE
To refine and validate a previously developed decision rule for obtaining ankle radiographs in acute ankle injuries.

METHODS
Two-stage, prospective, multicenter observational validation study in two Canadian academic EDs between 1991 and 1992. In the first stage, a previously derived decision rule was validated and refined. In the second stage, the refined rule was prospectively validated.

Patients
Convenience sample of patients with acute ankle pain from blunt trauma. 1,032 patients were enrolled in the first stage and 435 patients in the second stage. Patients were evaluated by two emergency physicians on 15 variables in the first stage, and 6 variables in the second. All patients then underwent radiography of the foot or ankle.

Intervention Evaluation
Standard radiographs of the foot or ankle to evaluate for significant fracture, defined as fractures with bone fragments greater than 3 mm.

Outcomes
The decision rule was evaluated for the ability to identify patients with high likelihood of negative radiography of the foot or ankle.

KEY RESULTS
- Five clinical criteria were identified as having the highest association with fracture. These resulted in the development of the Ottawa Foot and Ankle Rules:
  Radiographs are only indicated if patients present with one of the following:
  - Bone tenderness of the base of the fifth metatarsal

- Bone tenderness of the distal 6 cm of the posterior edge of the tibia or medial malleolus
- Bone tenderness of the distal 6 cm of the posterior edge of the fibula or the lateral malleolus
- Inability to bear weight and walk four steps both immediately and in the ED
- Bone tenderness at the navicular
• In the first stage, the decision rule was found to have a sensitivity of 100% for identifying fractures in the malleolar zone (ankle) and 98% for identifying fractures in the midfoot (navicular and fifth metatarsal).
• In the second stage, the revised decision rule was found to be 100% sensitive for identifying fractures in the malleolar zone and 100% for identifying fractures in the midfoot.
• The decision rule was predicted to reduce radiography of the ankle by 34% and of the foot by 30%.

STUDY CONCLUSIONS
The revised Ottawa Foot and Ankle Rules can rule out fractures of the ankle and midfoot with high sensitivity, potentially reducing unnecessary radiography in the ED.

COMMENTARY
This study derived a clinical decision rule that could be used to reliably identify patients presenting with acute ankle injuries who did not require radiographs as part of their ED evaluation. The Ottawa Ankle Rules have been validated in a number of populations and have become a mainstay of emergency medicine training and practice. The overall impact of this study has been limited, however, by a variety of factors including patient preference for x-rays. In addition, patients often describe ankle tenderness diffusely making it difficult to definitively say that patients have no tenderness within the loose definition of 6 cm of either malleolus. The Ottawa Foot and Ankle Rules, while likely underutilized, do offer clinicians a validated and sensitive method for identifying patients at low risk for acute fracture of the ankle or foot and laid the groundwork for many other clinical decision rules to guide care in the ED.

Question
Do all patients who present to the ED with acute ankle injuries require radiography to rule out a fracture?

Answer
No, the Ottawa Foot and Ankle Rules can identify patients at low risk for significant fracture, obviating the need for imaging.

SECTION 10
PAIN

Michael E. Billington

66. Morphine and the Clinical Abdominal Exam
67. Ketorolac vs. Ibuprofen in Musculoskeletal Pain
68. Pain Management in the ED: The PEMI Study

CHAPTER 66
MORPHINE AND THE CLINICAL ABDOMINAL EXAM

Randomized Clinical Trial of Morphine in Acute Abdominal Pain
Gallagher EJ, Esses D, Lee C, Lahn M, Bijur PE. *Ann Emerg Med.* 2006;48:150–160

BACKGROUND
Acute abdominal pain is the most common presenting complaint in EDs nationwide, accounting for more than 7 million visits annually. When encountered in the ED, a commonly heard phrase is "don't give opiates, it ruins the abdominal exam." For many years there had been conflicting consensus recommendations and a paucity of studies exploring the effect of treating acute abdominal pain in the ED with opiates. As such, many physicians were reluctant to treat pain due to the possibility of obscuring the diagnosis.

OBJECTIVES
To test the hypothesis that IV morphine given in the ED will improve, rather than diminish, diagnostic accuracy while simultaneously reducing patient discomfort.

METHODS
Randomized double-blind study in a US ED between 2002 and 2004.

Patients
One hundred and fifty-three patients, >21 years old, who presented with nontraumatic abdominal pain lasting less than 48 hours. Select exclusion criteria: patients who had taken or received analgesia prior to evaluation, patients presenting with isolated flank pain, sickle cell crisis, concurrent hypotension, or patients with an allergy to morphine.

Intervention Evaluated
After blinded dose of morphine 0.1 mg/kg or equivalent dose of normal saline (NS) was administered, an ED attending not involved in the patient's care performed an abdominal examination and provided a provisional diagnosis and disposition based on the examination. Patients in both groups were then eligible to receive opiate pain medications/antiemetics as needed.

Outcomes
The primary outcome was "clinically significant diagnostic accuracy" assessed at 6 weeks by two separate physician evaluators. This measure was the inverse of "clinically significant diagnostic error," which was defined as a difference in initial and final diagnosis that would have been expected to affect the patient's health. The secondary outcome was the accuracy of the provisional diagnosis.

KEY RESULTS
- Diagnostic accuracy was equivalent between the morphine and placebo groups (86% vs. 85%), with high interrater agreement at 99%.
- Disposition accuracies were similar and not statistically significant (58% vs. 55%).

STUDY CONCLUSIONS
Morphine administration for acute abdominal pain does not decrease the diagnostic accuracy of the physical examination.

COMMENTARY
At time of this publication the authors estimated that only one-fourth of patients with acute abdominal pain received morphine. However, these results demonstrate that emergency care providers can confidently treat pain in patients without fearing any decreased diagnostic accuracy. In addition to changing ED practice, this work also enabled emergency physicians to advocate for patient analgesia when communicating with consultants providing care and recommendations for patient in the ED. The findings of this work should be interpreted with some caution as more patients with a final diagnosis of nonspecific abdominal pain were randomized to the placebo arm by chance, which may have favored morphine treatment. Also this study only evaluated the use of initial opiate treatment and not multiple doses over the course of ED stay, so clinicians should bear caution when patients require escalating doses of analgesia with reassuring physical examinations. Regardless, this work supports the patient-centered treatment of acute abdominal pain with opiates, particularly in an era in which advanced radiography and laboratory tests have enabled prompter and more accurate diagnoses of abdominal disease.

Question
Can morphine be used to treat acute abdominal pain without obscuring the physical examination?

Answer
Yes, treating acute abdominal pain in the ED with opiate analgesia does not diminish diagnostic accuracy.

CHAPTER 67
KETOROLAC VS. IBUPROFEN IN MUSCULOSKELETAL PAIN

Intramuscular Ketorolac vs. Oral Ibuprofen in Acute Musculoskeletal Pain
Turturro MA, Paris PM, Seaberg DC. *Ann Emerg Med.* 1995;26(2):117–120

BACKGROUND
Ketorolac is the only parenteral (IV or IM) nonsteroidal anti-inflammatory (NSAID) and had been shown to provide similar relief when compared to one dose of selected opiates in nonemergent settings. Despite its benefit over opioids (including lack of respiratory depression, addiction potential, and sedation), it was unclear if there was any benefit over traditional oral NSAIDs such as ibuprofen for musculoskeletal pain. Traditional NSAIDs are significantly less costly than ketorolac.

OBJECTIVES
To compare the efficacy of oral ibuprofen to that of IM ketorolac in acute musculoskeletal pain in the ED.

METHODS
Randomized, prospective, double-blind, single-center trial in US ED.

Patients
Seventy-eight patients, 18 to 70 years old, with acute musculoskeletal pain after trauma. Select exclusion criteria: Patients with contraindications to NSAIDs, who had already taken a form of analgesia prior to arrival, or patients whom an ED physician felt required opioids due to severity of injury.

Intervention Evaluated
Patients were randomized to 60-mg IM ketorolac and placebo pill vs. 800-mg PO ibuprofen and IM normal saline injection.

Outcomes
Pain was evaluated by a visual analog scale (no pain 0 to worst pain imaginable 100) at baseline, 15, 30, 45, 60, 75, 90, and 120 minutes after dosing. Each patient was assessed for possible side effects.

KEY RESULTS
- No significant difference in pain control between IM ketorolac vs. PO ibuprofen from administration through 2 hours (mean pain at 2 hours, 33.5 in ketorolac group vs. 22.3 in ibuprofen, $p = 0.15$).
- Side effects were uncommon and not significant in either group.
- Five patients required opiates (two in ketorolac group vs. three in ibuprofen group, $p < 0.67$) because of inadequate pain control.

STUDY CONCLUSIONS
Single-dose ketorolac does not treat acute musculoskeletal pain better than single-dose ibuprofen in the ED.

COMMENTARY

Acute musculoskeletal pain makes up a large percentage of ED visits, and although previous studies showed similar efficacy between IM ketorolac when compared to opiates in pain syndromes such as renal colic, biliary colic, arthritis, postoperative pain, pharyngitis, and soft tissue trauma, this was the first study to compare the efficacy of PO vs. IM NSAIDS. This study showed no benefit to IM ketorolac over PO ibuprofen using a well-designed, robust double-blind randomized control trial. Because no difference in pain scores were achieved at multiple intervals up to 2 hours, this study allows the emergency physician to feel comfortable choosing less expensive (and less painful administration) of PO NSAIDs for acute musculoskeletal pain in the ED. A significant limitation of this study is that it excludes patients with acute back pain, a common ED musculoskeletal complaint. The generalizability of these findings may also be limited by the study's use of IM and not IV ketorolac, which is the route most often used. Also notable, was that both groups achieved a 50% reduction in pain at 2 hours showing the efficacy of non-opiate therapy for acute musculoskeletal pain in the ED.

Question
Is there any benefit to IM ketorolac compared to oral NSAIDs for the treatment of acute musculoskeletal pain?

Answer
No, ibuprofen is equally effective at reducing acute musculoskeletal pain in the ED.

CHAPTER 68
PAIN MANAGEMENT IN THE ED: THE PEMI STUDY

Pain the Emergency Department: Results of the Pain and Emergency Medicine Initiative (PEMI) Multicenter Study
Todd KH, Ducharme J, Choiniere M, et al. *J Pain.* 2007;8(6):460–466

BACKGROUND
Pain is the most common reason for presentation to an ED in the United States. Standardized pain assessment and reassessment along with education of patients regarding pain management are considered standard of care by the Joint Commission on Accreditation of Healthcare Organizations (JCAHO) statement of 2001. Despite this, at the time of this study it was not known whether these protocols were being applied and there was a concern that these simple interventions were not being done.

OBJECTIVES
To access the degree of compliance with the JCAHO recommendations regarding the assessment and reassessment of patients presenting to the ED with pain.

METHODS
Prospective, observational study conducted at 20 centers across the US and Canada.

Patients
Eight hundred and forty-two patients, 8 to 91 years old who presented across a convenience sample of three different 8-hour shifts with pain >3 on a 10-point scale. Select exclusion criteria: Patients who were intoxicated, altered, or if there was concern for cardiogenic chest pain.

Intervention Evaluated
Patient experience of pain in the ED was assessed by trained interviewers who asked patients about: (1) Pain intensity at the time of arrival and discharge from ED, (2) the patient's pain level after analgesia treatment (if given), and (3) the way the ED staff responded to their pain. These patients' charts were also evaluated for chief complaint, type of analgesia use, and final diagnosis. Documentation of pain assessment and reassessment by providers were also noted.

Outcomes
Primary outcomes included mean presenting pain score, change in severity of pain by time of discharge, time to analgesia administration, and percentage of charts with documentation of pain assessment and reassessment by providers. Secondary outcomes included percentage of patients who requested analgesia who actually received it and patient satisfaction about pain control.

KEY RESULTS
- Patients presented with a median pain score of 8 (4 to 10) and were discharged with a median pain score of 6 (0 to 10).
- Fifty percent (421) of patients had a meaningful (>2-point) reduction during their ED stay; 41% (353) reported "no improvement" or "worse" level of pain.
- Eighty-three percent (699) had a pain score documented; 31% (261) had one reassessment; 14% (118) had two reassessments.
- Of 70% (590) of patients who requested analgesia, only 60% (509) received it.
- Median time to analgesia administration is 90 minutes (0 to 962 minutes); only 29% (148) of patients were given medication within 1 hour of arrival.

STUDY CONCLUSIONS
Despite efforts to improve pain management in the ED, underutilization of pain medication and lack of adherence to standardized protocols remains a significant problem.

COMMENTARY
At the time of this study there was concern that ED patients were not being adequately treated for pain, yet no rigorous prospective studies had confirmed this hypothesis. This study prospectively examined and demonstrated that a large group of patients experience undertreated pain by multiple dimensions: Delayed therapy, inadequate pain reduction and reassessment, and most troublesome of all, a failure to administer analgesia to patients who requested pain treatment. These findings support provider efforts to improve their vigilance in asking patients with moderate-to-severe pain if they would like analgesia. While this work supports JCAHO compliance efforts, readers should note that all forms of analgesia were considered in this study as opposed to only opiates. Patient populations in which some analgesics may be contraindicated, especially geriatric patients and patient with known opiate abuse, likely contributed to a portion of patients under-treated for their pain. Subsequent clinical guidelines, national quality measures, and research have built on this work targeting the improvement of prompt analgesia with frequent reassessment across numerous populations in the ED.

Question
Is acute pain treated adequately in the ED?

Answer
No, emergency care providers have considerable opportunity to improve the timeliness, adequacy, and reassessment of pain in the ED.

SECTION 11
VENOUS THROMBOEMBOLISM

Fan Yang

69. Clinical Diagnosis of PE
70. Prospective Evaluation of the PERC
71. D-Dimer in DVT and PE
72. V/Q Scan in Acute PE: The Pioped Trial
73. CT Imaging for Acute PE: The PIOPED II Trial

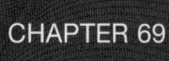

CHAPTER 69   CLINICAL DIAGNOSIS OF PE

Clinical Features From the History and Physical Examination That Predict the Presence or Absence of Pulmonary Embolism in Symptomatic Emergency Department Patients: Results of a Prospective, Multicenter Study
Courtney DM, Kline JA, Kabrhel C, et al. *Ann Emerg Med.* 2010;55(4):307–315

BACKGROUND
Pulmonary embolism (PE) is a disease with high mortality that is challenging to diagnose. Several pretest probability models utilize elements of history and physical examination (H&P) in predicting the likelihood of the diagnosis of PE, however, each individual H&P elements had yet to be validated in the ED setting. This study aimed to evaluate the soundness of various commonly used elements of H&P as predictors of diagnosis or exclusion of PE in large ED populations.

OBJECTIVE
To assess individual predictive values of 25 variables commonly used for the diagnosis of PE.

METHODS
Prospective, noninterventional, observational study, across 12 US centers (12 sites, nine teaching, and three community practices), between 2003 and 2006.

Participants
7,940 patients with signs and symptoms that warranted testing for PE. Select exclusion criteria: Suspicion of deep vein thrombosis (DVT) without PE, anticoagulation or inferior vena cava (IVC) filter, known DVT/PE, critical illness, homeless/incarcerated. All patients had either a D-dimer, CT Angiography (CTA), or Ventilation perfusion (V/Q) scan performed as a reference standard for the diagnosis of PE.

Intervention Evaluated
A survey with 25 predictors was provided to the treating physician. Responses regarding predictors that swayed the decision to test for PE were recorded. Of the 25 predictors, 12 were "explicit" predictors obtained from existing pretest probability models (Wells, revised Geneva, Charlotte, and PERC), and 13 were "implicit" predictors compiled through collective author experiences.

Outcomes
The primary outcome was diagnosis or treatment for PE or DVT within 45 days of index visit. Multivariate analysis was used to identify significant predictors of DVT/PE.

KEY RESULTS
- The most common complaints that lead to workup for DVT/PE were chest pain (71.8%) and dyspnea (70.4%).
- The three strongest predictors of PE were patient history of DVT/PE (OR = 2.9), unilateral leg swelling (OR = 2.6), and estrogen use (OR = 2.3). The strongest implicit predictor was personal history of noncancer-related thrombophilia (OR = 1.99).
- The three predictors that most negatively associated with diagnosis of PE were current smoking (OR = 0.59), substernal chest pain (OR = 0.58), and female sex (OR = 0.57).

STUDY CONCLUSIONS
Most clinical characteristics in existing clinical decision rules and several characteristics not currently included in these rules were significantly associated with a diagnosis of PE or DVT within 45 days.

COMMENTARY
The symptoms of PE are often vague and nonspecific, and this. This study provided the first prospective investigation in the ED of potential signs and symptoms that should elicit further diagnostic workup for PE. Unsurprisingly the cardinal symptoms of pleuritic chest pain and dyspnea are predictors for PE. The lack of association between sudden onset of symptoms, obesity, history of inactive malignancy, and fever are helpful in tipping the balance against testing for PE. Overall, this study confirms the difficulty of diagnosing or excluding PE based on H&P alone, and highlights the importance of utilizing validated structured pretest probability models.

Question
Can any single element of the history or physical examination predict the presence or absence of pulmonary embolism (PE)?

Answer
No, while individual history or physical examination elements cannot clinch the diagnosis of a PE; using multiple elements included in various structured decision rules can predict the presence or absence of a PE in the ED setting.

PROSPECTIVE EVALUATION OF THE PERC

Prospective Multicenter Evaluation of the Pulmonary Embolism Rule-out Criteria
Kline JA, Courtney DM, Kabrhel C, et al. *J Thromb Haemost.* 2008;6(5):772–780

BACKGROUND
Prior to this study, there were no validated clinical decision rules to identify a group at such low risk for pulmonary embolism (PE) that diagnostic testing could be omitted, limiting the risks of radiation, contrast dye exposure, and unnecessary anticoagulation. Existing validated clinical decision tools such as the Wells criteria allowed for low risk rule-out pathways without imaging, but did not obviate the need for laboratory testing. Previous attempts to validate the PERC rule did not yield satisfactory sensitivity, but they did not incorporate the application of clinical gestalt as a part of pre-test risk stratification prior to the application of PERC rules.

OBJECTIVE
To assess the validity of the PERC rule in a subset of patients judged to be at low risk of PE by clinical gestalt.

METHODS
Prospective, observational study of ED patients presenting to 12 centers in the United States and one in New Zealand between July 1, 2003 and November 30, 2006.

Patients
8,138 patients who had a diagnostic test ordered for PE (vascular imaging, ventilation perfusion (V/Q) scan, or D-dimer assay). Patients were enrolled in random 8-hour blocks consecutively at the discretion of the site. Eighty-five percent of patients had a presenting complaint of chest pain or dyspnea.

Data Collected
Prior to knowledge of testing results, the clinicians treating the patients filled out forms including their gestalt probability for PE prior to testing (low if <15%), the PERC components, and other clinical questions.

PULMONARY EMBOLISM RULE-OUT CRITERIA
- Low risk (<15%) by clinical gestalt (not previously included in other studies)
- Age <50
- HR <100
- SaO_2 >94% on room air
- No current hemoptysis
- No exogenous estrogen

- No history of venous thromboembolism
- No recent surgery (in the past 4 weeks, requiring endotracheal intubation or hospitalization)
- Absence of unilateral leg swelling

Outcomes
The primary outcome was venous thromboembolism (DVT or PE) at 45-day follow-up, plus documented intention to treat with at least 3 months of anticoagulation or a vena cava filter. Patients were defined as having PE if they had a high-probability V/Q scan, CT, or conventional angiogram interpreted as positive for PE, or an autopsy positive for PE. They were defined as having DVT if they had Doppler ultrasonography or CT venogram positive for acute femoral, axillary, or popliteal DVTs (not calf DVTs).

KEY RESULTS
- Twenty percent (1,666) of patients were classified as very low risk (low gestalt risk plus PERC negative).
- Per-site rates of patients at very low risk ranged from 10% to 36%.
- The false-negative rate of the PERC was 0. The articles false negative rate is 1.0%.
- PERC negative likelihood ratio was 0.12.
- The probability of PE after satisfying the PERC met the a priori goal of <2%.

STUDY CONCLUSIONS
The combination of low gestalt risk for PE and application of the PERC rule identified a subset of patients with less than a 1.0% chance of having a PE and for whom no workup should be performed as the risks of diagnosis outweigh the benefits.

COMMENTARY
This prospective validation of the PERC rule was pivotal in changing clinician's decision pathways when considering potential pulmonary emboli. The pretest probability of disease at which the risks of testing outweigh the benefits was determined to be 2%. Previous attempts to validate the PERC rule resulted in probabilities higher than this; the addition of low-risk gestalt to this validation attempt made the clinical use of the rule possible. It is critical in this context that clinicians avoid applying the PERC to high-risk patients. This study benefited from large samples from multiple centers as well as rigorous methodology. Placed in the increasingly relevant context of limited resource allocation, this study was one of the first to advocate a clinical decision rule which explicitly defines an acceptable miss rate (of about 1%). Application of this decision rule in an appropriately selected patient population has the potential to reduce resource utilization while simultaneously improving patient care by limiting radiation-induced malignancies, adverse reactions to contrast dye, and the risks of unnecessary anticoagulation.

Question

Does the PERC rule sufficiently exclude the diagnosis of pulmonary embolism?

Answer

Yes, while the PERC rule does not eliminate the possibility of a pulmonary embolism, it identifies a population for whom the risks of a diagnostic workup outweigh the benefits and for whom no further testing is necessary.

CHAPTER 71 D-DIMER IN DVT AND PE

D-dimer for the Exclusion of Acute Venous Thrombosis and Pulmonary Embolism: A Systematic Review

Stein PD, Hull RD, Patel KC, et al. *Ann Intern Med.* 2004;140(8):589–602

BACKGROUND
Since the 1980s a wide variety of D-dimer tests were studied for the exclusion of deep venous thrombosis (DVT) and pulmonary embolus (PE). The different tests reported widely varying accuracy. In the late 1990s, investigators attempted to establish unified recommendations regarding D-dimer testing but no consensus was reached, partially due to the variability of testing methodologies, identifying a need for a large scale review of the literature.

OBJECTIVE
To assess the accuracy of commonly used D-dimer assays in clinical practice.

METHODS
Systemic literature review of all published trials addressing the use of D-dimer to exclude PE or DVT between 1983 and 2003.

Inclusion Criteria
(1) Statement that PE or DVT was being diagnosed; (2) diagnosis of PE or DVT based on objective tests; (3) prospective studies; (4) consecutive recruitment; (5) broad-spectrum patient population; (6) independent interpretation of D-dimer and diagnostic tests for PE and DVT; (7) participants suspected of having PE or DVT; (8) reference diagnostic test decision made independently of the D-dimer result; (9) detailed test descriptions permit replication; (10) negative D-dimer cutoff value stated unless qualitative tests were used; and (11) sensitivity and specificity presented.

Patients
One hundred and forty-four articles were included.

Outcomes
Sensitivity, specificity, positive likelihood ratio (PLR), and negative likelihood ratio (NLR) of D-dimer testing, for detection of DVT and PE were calculated.

KEY RESULTS
- For detection of DVT, ELISA and quantitative rapid ELISA provided the best sensitivity (0.96 and 0.96) and NLR (0.12 and 0.09).
- For detection of PE, ELISA and quantitative rapid ELISA provided the best sensitivity (0.95 and 0.95) and NLR (0.13 and 0.13).
- Whole blood agglutination test provided the best specificity (0.87 for DVT and 0.74 for PE) but poor sensitivity.

STUDY CONCLUSION
ELISA and quantitative rapid ELISA provide clear superiority over other D-dimer assays and high sensitivity for the exclusion of DVT and PE.

COMMENTARY
Prior to this review, significant variability existed in types of D-dimer assays used and reported sensitivity and specificity related to D-dimer testing for exclusion of DVT/PE. As a result of this variability, clinicians had varying degrees of belief in the meaningfulness of D-dimer results in the evaluation of patients with suspected venous thromboembolism. This review clearly demonstrated the superiority of ELISA/quantitative ELISA over older assays with superior NLRs and higher sensitivity. The NLRs reported in this study are similar to those of near normal V/Q scan for detection of PE (NLR 0.10) and compression ultrasound (NLR 0.07) for detection of DVT. When applied alongside structured pretest probability assessment tools such as the Wells criteria, D-dimer has become widely used to rule out PE in the ED.

Question
Can the use of D-dimer testing exclude the diagnosis of DVT/PE?

Answer
Yes, use of a high-sensitivity D-dimer assay, particularly a quantitative ELISA, has high sensitivity and negative predictive value for excluding DVT/PE in patients with a low pretest probability.

CHAPTER 72
V/Q SCAN IN ACUTE PE: THE PIOPED TRIAL

Value of the Ventilation/Perfusion Scan in Acute Pulmonary Embolism: Results of the Prospective Investigation of Pulmonary Embolism Diagnosis (PIOPED)
PIOPED Investigators. *JAMA.* 1990;263(20):2753–2759

BACKGROUND
In the 1980s, pulmonary angiography was the gold standard imaging modality for the diagnosis of pulmonary embolism (PE). However, it was resource intensive, requiring skilled angiographer and specialized facilities, and invasive. Lack of access to testing resulted in many missed PEs with significant preventable mortality. Ventilation and perfusion lung scans (V/Q scan) was an emerging noninvasive alternative, showing some diagnostic value, but had not yet been validated in large populations. The PIOPED investigators sought to validate V/Q scan as a reliable diagnostic method for the diagnosis of PE.

OBJECTIVE
To determine the sensitivity and specificity of V/Q lung scan for diagnosis of PE.

METHODS
Prospective, multicenter, observational study conducted at six hospitals between 1985 and 1986.

Participants
933 patients, >18 years old, with symptoms suggestive of PE and the ability to obtain the study within 24 hours were included. Select exclusion criteria: pregnancy, elevated creatinine, contrast allergy, or other contraindications to angiography.

Intervention Evaluated
Patients underwent V/Q scan as well as the reference standard study (pulmonary angiography). V/Q findings were categorized as high, intermediate, low, and near normal/normal probability. Pretest clinical suspicion was recorded based on physician judgment.

Outcomes
Normal/near normal V/Q scan virtually excluded PE and high-probability V/Q scans were highly specific for PE, but intermediate results did not offer diagnostic certainty. Combining clinical assessment with concordant V/Q scan interpretation improved diagnostic yield.

KEY RESULTS
- The majority of V/Q scans had intermediate or low probability readings (39% and 34%, respectively).

- Near normal/normal V/Q scans (14% of scans done) had sensitivity of 98% and specificity of 10% for diagnosis of PE.
- High-probability V/Q scans (13% of scans done) had sensitivity of 41% and specificity of 97%.
- Patients with high clinical probability of PE and high-probability V/Q scan had a high likelihood of having a PE (positive predictive value 95%) whereas patients with low clinical probability of PE and low-probability V/Q scan had low likelihood of PE (negative predictive value 96%).

STUDY CONCLUSION

V/Q scans that are of high probability usually indicate PE, whereas near normal/normal scans exclude PE. In combination with pretest clinical impression, V/Q scans provide for a noninvasive method of diagnosis or exclusion of PE in a minority of patients in the study.

COMMENTARY

Prior to PIOPED, pulmonary angiogram was the gold standard diagnostic modality for PE, but its invasive nature, lack of availability, and resource intensiveness limited its practicality as a screening tool to rule out PE in the ED. V/Q scans showed promise, and PIOPED was the first large scale study investigating its reliability compared directly to angiography. The results showed that unequivocal V/Q scans were of high diagnostic accuracy, with the caveat that most patients had intermediate scans that did not provide a definitive diagnosis. Lesions from PIOPED led to the development of clinical algorithms incorporating pretest risk stratification with clinical decision rules (e.g., Wells criteria), laboratory studies such as D-dimer and definitive imaging to both reduce the need for extraneous studies and enhance the diagnostic yield of studies obtained. PIOPED was the first step in the transition toward the use of noninvasive imaging for diagnosis of PE.

Question
Can a V/Q scan be used to exclude the diagnosis of pulmonary embolism?

Answer
Yes, a normal V/Q scan can safely exclude the diagnosis of pulmonary embolism in patients with a low pretest probability.

CHAPTER 73
CT IMAGING FOR ACUTE PE: THE PIOPED II TRIAL

Multidetector Computed Tomography for Acute Pulmonary Embolism
Stein PD, Fowler SE, Goodman LR, et al. *NEJM.* 2006;354(22):2317–2327

BACKGROUND
Pulmonary embolism (PE) is associated with significant mortality and can pose a diagnostic challenge in the ED. In the early 2000s, ventilation/perfusion scan (V/Q scan) and pulmonary angiography were the primary modalities for the diagnosis of PE. Early single-slice CT had sensitivities ranging from 60% to 100%, but an inability to reliably assess segmental and subsegmental pulmonary arteries limited the ability to rule out PE. Multislice computed tomographic angiography (CTA) emerged as a novel, rapid, and noninvasive alternative, but its diagnostic accuracy was unknown. The PIOPED II study evaluated the reliability CTA for detection of acute PE in broad populations of patients spanning the inpatient, outpatient, and ED setting.

OBJECTIVE
To determine whether CTA, with and without the addition of computed tomographic venous-phase imaging (CTV), could reliably detect and rule out PE.

METHODS
Prospective, observation study across eight centers, between 2001 and 2003.

Participants
1,090 patients, >18 years old with clinical suspicion of acute PE. Eight hundred and twenty-four patients received a reference diagnostic test and CTA, most with low or moderate pretest probability of PE. Select exclusion criteria: Inability to complete testing within 36 hours, elevated creatinine, anticoagulated, critically ill, MI within preceding month, cardiac arrest, planned thrombolytic therapy, inferior vena cava (IVC) filter, upper extremity deep vein thrombosis (DVT), and pregnancy.

Intervention Evaluated
CTA and CTA-CTV compared to a composite reference standard (pulmonary angiography, V/Q scan, or venous compression ultrasound of lower extremities). Criteria for exclusion of acute PE by reference standard included one of the following findings: Normal, low, or very low probability for PE on V/Q scan, normal venous ultrasonography, normal pulmonary angiography, or Wells score less than 2.

Outcomes
Primary outcomes were the sensitivity and specificity of CTA for diagnosis of PE and the impact of the addition of CTV in diagnosis. The secondary outcome was the impact of using a pretest risk stratification with the Wells criteria when combined with CTA and CTV.

KEY RESULTS
- CTA has 83% sensitivity and 96% specificity for detection of acute PE.
- Addition of CTV improved sensitivity to 90% while maintaining similar specificity 95%.
- High clinical probability Wells criteria improved CTA *positive* predictive value to 96% while low probability Wells criteria improved CTA *negative* predictive value to 97%.
- For the majority of patients with intermediate clinical probability of PE, CTA had negative predictive value of 89%. The addition of CTV only marginally improved predictive values after clinical preassessment was applied.

STUDY CONCLUSION
In patients with suspected PE, the sensitivity of CTA or CTA-CTV is high, and improved when combined with a high probability Wells score.

COMMENTARY
Rapid and accurate diagnosis of PE is a challenge in the ED. While the gold standard, the pulmonary angiogram is highly sensitive and specific, it is an invasive and technically difficult procedure. The advent of V/Q scanning paved the way for noninvasive testing but produced many indeterminate findings that complicated clinical decision making. This study confirmed that CTA is a reliable and accurate tool for the diagnosis or exclusion of PE that is rapid and broadly effective across a large multicenter trial. Since this study, there has been near universal adoption of CTA as the gold standard imaging tool for the diagnosis of PE. The 17% false negative rate was higher than expected, but subsequent outcome studies have demonstrated the safety of withholding treatment in patients with low and intermediate Wells criteria who have negative CTA studies, making this less of a concern. While CTA-CTV has more sensitivity than CTA alone, the improvement is marginal especially when pretest clinical assessment is taken into account. PIOPED II firmly establishes the role of CTA as an accurate first-line imaging modality for diagnosis of PE and reaffirms the importance of incorporating clinical preassessment with diagnostic imaging for the exclusion and diagnosis of PE.

Question
Can CT angiography safely exclude the diagnosis of pulmonary embolism?

Answer
Yes, when concordant with Wells criteria, multidetector CT angiography improves diagnostic accuracy for acute PE.

SECTION 12
PSYCHIATRY

Daphne Morrison Ponce

74. Pharmaceutical Restraints for Psychotic Agitation

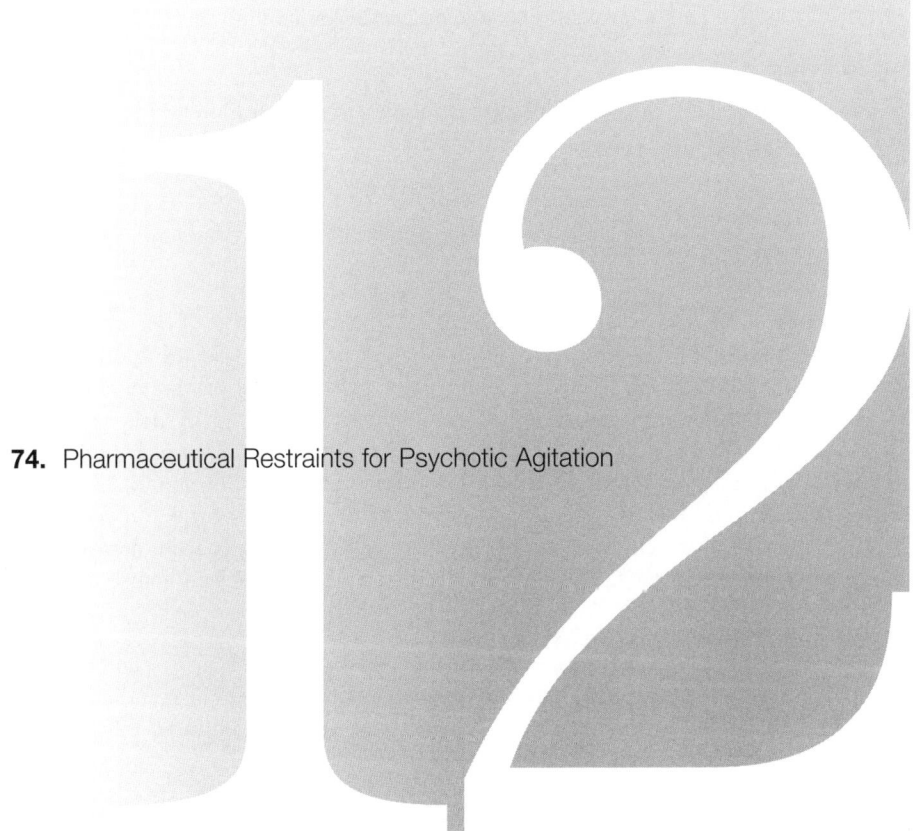

CHAPTER 74: PHARMACEUTICAL RESTRAINTS FOR PSYCHOTIC AGITATION

Haloperidol, Lorazepam or Both for Psychotic Agitation? A Multicenter, Prospective, Double-blind, Emergency Department Study
Battaglia J, Moss S, Rush J, et al. *Am J Emerg Med.* 1997;15(4):335–340

BACKGROUND
Haloperidol has been used in escalating doses to control agitated psychotic patients, reduce assaults, and decrease the need for physical restraints. In practice, low-dose antipsychotics are often combined with lorazepam, or other benzodiazepines, for better behavioral control. At the time of this study prior trials had evaluated this practice but had limitations in study design: unblinded investigators, minimal measurement of drug adverse effects, and had no evaluation of the patient beyond falling asleep the first time.

OBJECTIVES
To prospectively evaluate the clinical response of patients in an ED to rapid tranquilization (RT) using either lorazepam or haloperidol, or both in combination.

METHODS
Prospective, randomized controlled trial at five different hospital emergency rooms over an 18-month period.

Participants
Ninety-eight patients who exhibited psychosis and behavior dyscontrol, and scored greater than a 5 on a seven-point Brief Psychiatric Rating Scale. All patients meeting the inclusion criteria were included regardless of underlying etiology of their symptoms. However, patients who were clinically intoxicated with alcohol were not included due to the risk of respiratory depression with the addition of a benzodiazepine. Key exclusion criteria: central nervous system (CNS) depression, delirium, neuroleptic malignant syndrome, airway obstruction, severe hypotension or hypertension, acute narrow angle glaucoma, and treatment with the study medication in the previous 24 hours.

Intervention Evaluated
Patients were computed randomized to receive haloperidol, lorazepam, or combination therapy. Both patients and physicians were blinded to the treatment arm. Patients could get redosed as needed within the first 12 hours and then were monitored for 24 hours. Initial doses were given every 60 minutes as needed.

Outcomes
The primary outcome was efficacy as assessed on the Agitated Behavior Scale (ABS), a modified Brief Psychiatric Rating Scale, Clinical Global Impressions Scale, and an Alertness Scale.

KEY RESULTS
- All treatment groups showed reduced ABS scores from baseline; however, patients in the combination group showed significantly greater reduction in ABS score than those receiving lorazepam alone.
- The combination group had lower ABS scores than the haloperidol alone group; however, this was not significant.
- The combination group also showed statistically significant improvement at hours 2 and 3. There were no differences in the single-agent treatment groups.
- The potential drug side effects were similar among the three groups.

STUDY CONCLUSIONS
Combination therapy of lorazepam and haloperidol is superior to single-agent therapy for acute psychotic agitation.

COMMENTARY
The acutely psychotic patient presents a challenge to emergency physicians, posing a safety risk to the patient, staff, and others in the ED. This study demonstrates that combination haloperidol and lorazepam provides better sedation and behavioral control without increased risk of side effects, laying the groundwork for what is now the standard of care. Note that this study was small and excluded patients who were already sedated or acutely intoxicated with alcohol, and thus is not generalizable to these populations that frequently present with acute agitation. Also, the small sample size risks being underpowered to detect all adverse outcomes. While this study only carries a Level C recommendation in clinical practice guidelines, the use of dual therapy for acute agitation has become routine across US EDs.

Question
Should haloperidol or lorazepam be used in isolation when treating a psychotic patient in the ED posing a danger to staff and to him/herself?

Answer
No, in patients who are not clinically intoxicated, the combination therapy of haloperidol (5 mg) and lorazepam (2 mg) is more effective at decreasing agitation than either agent alone.

SECTION 13: PULMONARY

Radhika Sundararajan ■ Joshua M. Keegan

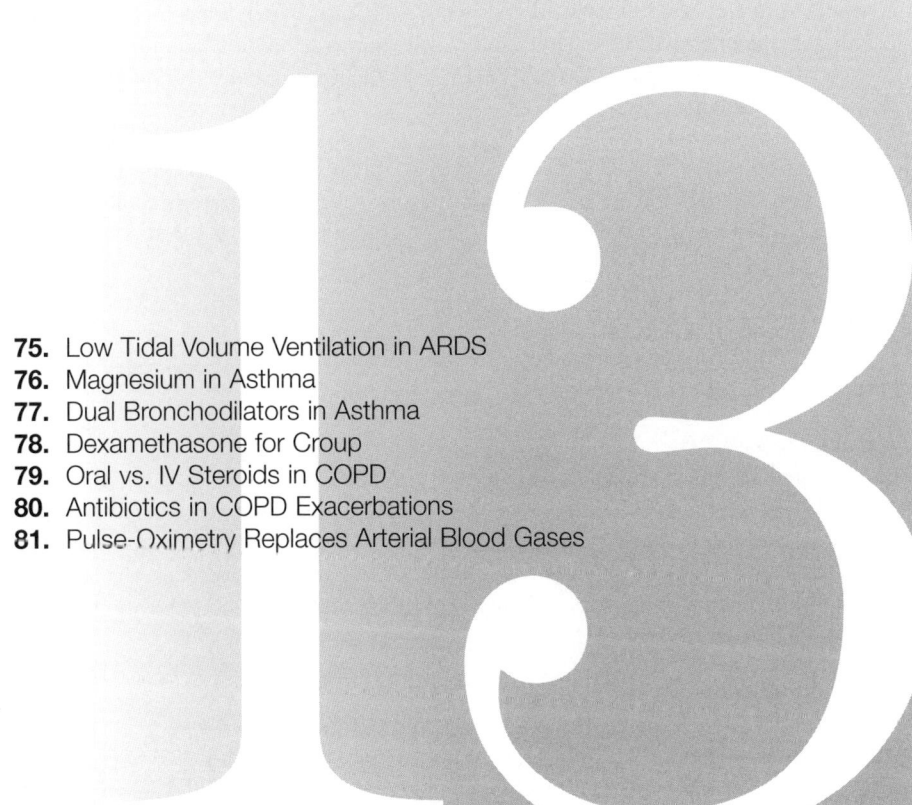

75. Low Tidal Volume Ventilation in ARDS
76. Magnesium in Asthma
77. Dual Bronchodilators in Asthma
78. Dexamethasone for Croup
79. Oral vs. IV Steroids in COPD
80. Antibiotics in COPD Exacerbations
81. Pulse-Oximetry Replaces Arterial Blood Gases

CHAPTER 75
LOW TIDAL VOLUME VENTILATION IN ARDS

Ventilation With Lower Tidal Volumes as Compared With Traditional Tidal Volumes for Acute Lung Injury and the Acute Respiratory Distress Syndrome
The Acute Respiratory Distress Syndrome Network. *N Engl J Med.* 2000;342(18):1301–1308

BACKGROUND
Acute lung injury and acute respiratory distress syndrome (ARDS) have high associated mortality. At the time of this study, it was posited that ventilation strategies using high tidal volumes (10 to 15 cc/kg) could lead to lung distention that exacerbate lung injury and ARDS. It was thought that lower tidal volume ventilation could reduce lung injury but would result in respiratory acidosis, hypoxemia, and hypercarbia. At the time of the study, it was unknown whether a high tidal volume or low tidal volume ventilation strategy was superior in patients with ARDS and the risks of conventional ventilation had not been studied.

OBJECTIVES
To determine whether the use of a low tidal volume ventilation strategy could improve outcomes in patients with ARDS by comparing high vs. low tidal volume ventilation patients.

METHODS
Prospective, multicenter, randomized trial at 10 tertiary academic medical centers between March 1996 and March 1999.

Participants
861 intubated and mechanically ventilated adult patients with ARDS, defined as ratio of partial pressure of arterial oxygen to fraction of inspired oxygen (P/f ratio) of less than 300 mm Hg or bilateral pulmonary infiltrates on chest radiography were included. Select exclusion criteria: Known severe chronic respiratory disease, sickle cell, severe burns, morbid obesity, or other preexisting conditions with an estimated 6-month mortality rate of 50% or higher.

Intervention Evaluated
Low tidal volume ventilation strategy, which used tidal volumes of 4 to 6 cc/kg, maximum plateau pressures of 30 cm H_2O, with bicarbonate infusions allowed to correct for acidosis. This was compared to high tidal volume strategy which used tidal volumes of 10 to 12 cc/kg and maximum plateau pressure of 45 to 50 cm of H_2O. Patients were monitored for 28 days.

Outcomes
Primary outcomes were (1) Death before discharge home and breathing without assistance at 180 days and (2) Number of days without ventilator use during the first 28 days. Data was also collected on arterial pH and partial pressures of oxygen and carbon dioxide, serum interleukin 6 (IL-6) levels, and signs of organ or systemic failure.

KEY RESULTS
- The trial was stopped early after 861 patients because mortality was lower in the lower tidal volume treatment group (31% vs. 39.8%) and days without ventilator assistance were greater (12 vs. 10).
- Mean tidal volumes and plateau pressures were 6.2 cc/kg and 25 cm H_2O respectively in the low tidal volume group and 11.8 cc/kg and 33 cm H_2O in the high tidal volume group.
- Number of days without nonpulmonary organ failure was higher in the lower tidal volume group but the incidence of barotrauma was similar between groups.

STUDY CONCLUSIONS
Lower tidal volume ventilation strategy yielded a mortality benefit, more ventilator-free days, and reduced nonpulmonary organ failure in patients with ARDS.

COMMENTARY
This is a landmark, large, multicenter, prospective, randomized trial showing a significant mortality benefit from low tidal volume ventilation in patients with ARDS, a disease that formerly had almost no effective therapies. Key to the trial's positive results was the fact that the investigators used a very low starting tidal volume that was calculated using predicted body weight rather than actual body weight (thus increasing the difference between groups and minimizing tidal volumes in the experimental group). They found no differences in gross barotrauma (mostly pneumothorax) between study groups. Patients in the low tidal volume group had notably lower plateau pressures, higher PEEP, and lower levels of inflammatory markers, hence investigators postulate that reduction in microalveolar, atelectotrauma may be responsible for some of the benefit, a theory that has been supported by subsequent study. The authors also tried to limit survival bias in the study by excluding patients with morbid conditions (transplant, severe respiratory disease, cirrhosis, or morbid obesity), however, this limits generalizability of the study findings to a healthier cohort of ARDS patients.

Question
Are there any specific mechanical ventilation settings that improve outcomes in patients with acute respiratory distress syndrome (ARDS)?

Answer
Yes, low tidal volume ventilation provides a mortality benefit without increasing adverse events in mechanically ventilated adult patients with ARDS.

CHAPTER 76: MAGNESIUM IN ASTHMA

Intravenous Magnesium as an Adjuvant in Acute Bronchospasm: A Meta-Analysis
Alter HJ, Koepsell TD, Hilty WM. *Ann Emerg Med.* 2000;36(3):191–197

BACKGROUND
It is estimated that 5% to 10% of all patients with asthma will present with an acute exacerbation that does not respond to typical bronchodilator therapy. This is a major cause of morbidity and the source of 440,000 annual hospitalizations with an average length of stay of 3.6 days. In vitro studies have shown that magnesium has bronchodilating capacity through smooth muscle relaxation that operates independently of the beta-2 receptor. Studies prior to 2000 showed conflicting results on the benefit of IV magnesium in acute asthma exacerbation. Prior to this meta-analysis little was known about the efficacy of IV Magnesium in the ED treatment of acute asthma and chronic obstructive pulmonary disease (COPD) exacerbations.

OBJECTIVES
To determine whether the addition of IV magnesium bolus to standard therapy improves acute bronchospasm.

METHODS
Meta-analysis of nine clinical trials.

Patients
Eight hundred and fifty-nine patients from nine studies were included. Inclusion criteria were acute bronchospasm, either due to asthma or COPD, presenting to an ED or acute care setting. Severity of illness measurements varied from FEV1 <75% to peak expiratory flow rate (PEFR) <30% of predicted. Both adults and children were included. Select exclusion criteria: Oral or continuous infusion of magnesium. Patients with only mild exacerbations (patients who did not require IV steroids, or whose respiratory status improved with three nebulized bronchodilator treatments) were also excluded.

Interventions
Randomized controlled trials of IV magnesium vs. placebo as adjuvant to standard treatment of acute bronchospasm in ED or acute care settings were included in this study. All but one of the studies was double-blinded. A specific dose of IV magnesium was not standardized between the studies (doses ranged from 10 mg/kg to 2 g).

Outcomes
Primary outcome was PEFR. No secondary outcomes were considered.

KEY RESULTS
- IV magnesium resulted in improved PEFR by 16% (summary effect size of 0.162).
- The pooled standard deviation of PEFR in the studies was 101 L/min (or improvement of approximately 16 L/min).
- No major adverse events were reported from any of the studies.

STUDY CONCLUSIONS
IV magnesium is a low-cost and safe therapy that should be considered as an adjuvant treatment for patients with moderate to severe bronchospasm.

COMMENTARY
Prior to this study there was conflicting evidence on the effectiveness of magnesium in asthma and COPD exacerbation. Widespread use by clinicians of this medication was prompted by the fact that they had few pharmacologic options and high morbidity and mortality associated with this disease. This study attempted to apply common principles of evaluation to existing data, and showed that IV magnesium was an effective, safe, and low-cost intervention. This conclusion was confirmed by a subsequent meta-analysis in a subset of patients with PEFR <25% of expected. However, the summary statistic the authors used was predicated on the assumption of no between-study variation, which is unlikely, as the included studies varied widely with regard to mean age, magnesium regimen, treatment of bronchospasm, and use of steroids. Using a more realistic model (which considers variability between studies), the results of the meta-analysis are not statistically significant. As such, current guidelines only favor the use of IV magnesium in those patients with severe exacerbation and objective evidence of bronchospasm.

Question
Does magnesium improve outcomes in patients with acute bronchospasm?

Answer
Yes, IV magnesium is a safe and inexpensive adjuvant intervention that improves pulmonary function in severe exacerbations.

CHAPTER 77
DUAL BRONCHODILATORS IN ASTHMA

Nebulized Salbutamol With and Without Ipratropium Bromide in the Treatment of Acute Asthma
Garrett JE, Town GI, Rodwell P, Kelly AM. *J Allergy Clin Immunol.* 1997;100(2):165–170

BACKGROUND
Asthma has a wide clinical spectrum ranging from mild to life-threatening disease. While deaths due to asthma exacerbation are rare (1/2,000 asthmatics), they have been increasing worldwide. Prior to this study, anticholinergic medications were used in ambulatory and ED settings despite a lack of clinical evidence to support the addition of nebulized ipratropium to beta-agonist nebulizers. Several prior studies had suggested a benefit, but were too small to show statistically significant outcomes.

OBJECTIVES
To determine if single dose ipratropium, in addition to nebulized beta-agonists, improves outcomes for ED patients presenting with acute asthma exacerbation.

METHODS
Double-blind, randomized trial across two EDs in New Zealand.

Participants
Three hundred and thirty-eight patients with acute asthma exacerbation. Mean age for both groups was approximately 29 years old, with approximately 32% active smokers and pulmonary functions tests (PFTs) notable for 39% of predicted FEV_1 in both groups. Select exclusion criteria: >10 pack-year smoking history, "complicating medical diseases" (chronic obstructive pulmonary disease, pneumonia, pneumothorax, congestive heart failure, acute renal insufficiency, or hepatic insufficiency), or pregnant or breast-feeding women.

Intervention Evaluated
A single dose of nebulized 2.5 mg salbutamol or 0.5 mg ipratropium/2.5 mg salbutamol was administered. All patients also received 200 mg IV hydrocortisone within 15 minutes of treatment initiation. No other medications were administered unless deemed necessary by the treating ED physician, at which point patients were removed from the study after measurement of final FEV_1.

Outcomes
Primary end point was FEV_1 at 90 minutes, using intention to treat analysis.

KEY RESULTS
- The ipratropium plus salbutamol group showed an improvement in FEV_1 at 45 minutes (93 ± 24 mL, $p = 0.03$) and 90 minutes (113 ± 18 mL, $p = 0.02$)

compared with salbutamol alone. The addition of ipratropium did not have any negative hemodynamic effects on heart rate or blood pressure.
- Patients with more severe disease (defined as lower FEV_1) and those who had consumed the highest amounts of beta-agonist prior to ED presentation were less likely to improve with either treatment, and did not show benefit with addition of ipratropium.
- The study was powered adequately to detect a 0.05 level of significance with a 150 mL difference in FEV_1 between the two treatment arms with 90% probability. While the maximum difference in FEV_1 observed was less than this (113 mL), this improvement was still statistically significant.

STUDY CONCLUSIONS
One dose of ipratropium augments the effects of salbutamol and produces statistically significant improvement in FEV_1. However, this benefit may not translate to patients with severe disease or who have consumed large amounts of beta-agonist within 6 hours of ED presentation.

COMMENTARY
The use of anticholinergic medication in the treatment of acute asthma exacerbation was fairly widespread in ambulatory and ED settings, despite a lack of strong clinical evidence to support this practice. This study was designed and powered effectively to demonstrate that the addition of an anticholingeric agent to beta-agonists is safe and beneficial in improving pulmonary function for patients with acute asthma exacerbation. The primary challenge in interpreting these findings is the use of FEV_1 as a primary end point. This physiologic variable is often measured by pulmonologists, but is not correlated with decreased need for intubation, fewer hospital days, or even improvement in peak flow, the latter being a variable more commonly measured and used in the ED as a marker for clinical improvement. Also of note, albuterol use in the prehospital setting might have varied between the two treatment groups as 80% had received beta-agonists within 6 hours of ED evaluation, which may have moderated the effects of beta-agonists on more meaningful outcomes that clinically seem apparent such as reduced dyspnea, hospitalization, and intubation. Based on this study and subsequent work, the initial use of combination bronchodilators has become standard in asthma treatment protocols and guidelines.[1]

Question
Does the addition of ipratropium to albuterol improve outcomes in patients with acute asthma exacerbations?

Answer
Yes, combination therapy improves pulmonary function without any notable adverse events; however, the impact on clinical outcomes such as intubation or hospital length of stay remains unclear.

Reference
1. 2007 guidelines for diagnosis and management of asthma by NHLBI. http://www.nhlbi.nih.gov/guidelines/asthma/asthsumm.pdf

CHAPTER 78
DEXAMETHASONE FOR CROUP

A Randomized Trial of a Single Dose of Oral Dexamethasone for Mild Croup
Bjornson CL, Klassen TP, Williamson J, et al. *N Engl J Med.* 2004;351(13):1306–1313

BACKGROUND
Croup is a common illness in children, and a common presentation in the ED. The majority of children with croup have a mild course, with a minority of patients requiring hospitalization or endotracheal intubation. Corticosteroids have proven beneficial in the treatment of moderate to severe croup but at the time of this study their efficacy in mild croup was unknown.

OBJECTIVES
To determine whether a single dose of dexamethasone for children with mild croup reduces the return to a medical provider, as well as associated economic costs.

METHODS
Multicenter, randomized, double-blind, placebo-controlled trial in four Canadian pediatric EDs between 2001 and 2003.

Participants
Seven hundred and twenty children who displayed symptoms of "mild croup" (defined as onset within 72 hours of barking cough and a Croup Score of 2 or less out of 17). Select exclusion criteria: Alternative diagnosis of stridor (supraglottic foreign body, epiglottitis), history of congenital or acquired stridor, exposure to corticosteroid in the past 2 weeks, immunosuppression, or non-English speaking parents.

Intervention Evaluated
Each child received a single dose of dexamethasone (0.6 mg/kg) or placebo (distilled water) orally. Both were mixed with cherry-flavored syrup and not distinguishable by weight, smell, or appearance.

Outcomes
Primary outcome was return to a health care provider within 7 days. Secondary outcomes included presence of ongoing croup symptoms on days 1, 2, and 3 after treatment, costs to child's family and "payer" (Canadian provincial government in this case) in 21 days following treatment, hours of sleep missed by the child, and stress experienced by the parent due to the illness.

KEY RESULTS
- Return to health care provider within 7 days was significantly higher among placebo vs. corticosteroid groups (15% vs. 7%), with adjusted OR 2.4. The number needed to treat to prevent one return visit was 13.
- The corticosteroid group showed benefit among all secondary outcomes, including lower costs, less sleep lost, and decreased parental stress on day 1. However, parental stress scores were not different between groups on days 2 and 3 of illness.
- Ongoing symptoms were more pronounced in the placebo group within the first 24 hours of treatment, but the two groups were nearly identical with regard to symptom severity on day 3 following treatment.

STUDY CONCLUSIONS
This study shows benefit of dexamethasone treatment for children with mild croup. These benefits extend across clinical, social, and economic outcome measures.

COMMENTARY
Mild croup rarely results in adverse clinical outcomes, but the social and economic effect of illness can be severe for children and their families, including lost sleep, and time away from school or work. Very little research had previously focused on patient-centered outcomes such as these. These data show that a single dose of dexamethasone—a simple and inexpensive intervention—has benefit across clinical, economic, and social outcomes. As mild croup is a more common presentation than moderate or severe disease, this study is applicable to the majority of croup patients evaluated in EDs. Of note, the use of corticosteroids does not impact morbidity and mortality, but improved costs and quality of life are statistically significant with only a single dose in the ED. The efficacy of a single dose of dexamethasone was validated by a subsequent Cochrane analysis[1] and is now considered the mainstay of treating croup in ambulatory and ED settings.

Question
Do steroids improve outcomes in children presenting with acute croup?

Answer
Yes, children with mild croup treated with a single dose of dexamethasone are more likely to have improved symptoms within 24 hours and less likely to return to a medical provider in seven days.

Reference
1. Russell KF, Liang Y, O'Gorman K, et al. Glucocorticoids for croup. *Cochrane Database Syst Rev.* 2011;(1).

CHAPTER 79
ORAL VS. IV STEROIDS IN COPD

Oral or Intravenous Prednisolone in the Treatment of COPD Exacerbations: A Randomized Controlled, Double Blind Study

de Jong YP, Uil SM, Grotjohan HP, Postma DS, Kerstjens HA, van den Berg JW. Chest. 2007;132(6):1741–1747

BACKGROUND
Chronic obstructive pulmonary disease (COPD) is a major health problem worldwide, with exacerbations being a frequent cause for ED presentation and hospitalization. While systemic corticosteroids have long been a crucial component in the treatment of COPD exacerbations, the ideal route of administration was not known. IV corticosteroid preparations were more often used based on the theoretical concern around the PO delayed onset of action, however, are more costly and difficult to administer. At the time of this study, no evidence existed comparing the efficacy of oral and IV routes of corticosteroid administration.

OBJECTIVES
To determine if oral prednisolone is not inferior to IV prednisolone in treatment of patients hospitalized with COPD exacerbations.

METHODS
Randomized, double-blind trial at one hospital center between 2001 and 2003.

Patients
Two hundred and ten patients admitted for COPD exacerbations. Select exclusion criteria: "Severe exacerbation" (arterial pH <7.26, $PaCO_2$ >9.3 kPa), "significant or unstable comorbidity" (not further defined), patients with known history of asthma, or patients with chest radiograph findings suggesting another diagnosis in addition to COPD, such as pneumonia.

Intervention Evaluated
Patients were randomized to either receive a 5-day course of IV or oral prednisolone (60 mg). All patients were transitioned to oral taper after 5 days, and concurrently treated with albuterol/ipratropium nebulizers QID as well as oral amoxicillin/clavulanate (doxycycline for those with allergy).

Outcomes
The primary outcome was treatment failure, defined as death from any cause, admission to the ICU, readmission due to COPD exacerbation, or need to add medications to standard treatment (including theophylline, open-label corticosteroids or antibiotics). Treatment failure was divided into early (within first 2 weeks) vs. late (from 2 weeks to

3 months). Secondary end points included improvements in FEV_1 between days 1 and 7, SGRQ scores (St. George Respiratory Questionnaire), CCQ score (Clinical COPD Questionnaire), and length of hospital stay.

KEY RESULTS
- There was no significant difference in treatment failure rates between oral and IV groups (56.3% vs. 61.7% at 90 days)
- Comparison of total, early and late treatment failure between two groups showed noninferiority of oral prednisolone.
- There was no statistical difference in any secondary end points. Length of hospitalization was slightly (but not significantly) shorter among patients undergoing oral therapy (11.9 ± 8.6 vs. 11.2 ± 6.7).

STUDY CONCLUSION
Orally administered prednisolone is not inferior to IV administered prednisolone in clinical treatment of COPD exacerbation. This should therefore be the preferred route, as it is less expensive and does not carry risk of infection.

COMMENTARY
This study demonstrated noninferiority of oral steroids for patients presenting with COPD exacerbation. This suggests the oral route is preferable for patients who are able to tolerate oral medication, as oral treatment is not only less costly but may also be able to avoid painful or challenging IV placement in some patients with mild exacerbations. One study limitation worth considering was that the IV treatment group received 60 mg prednisolone, which is equivalent to 48 mg IV methylprednisolone (the more commonly used dose of methylprednisolone is 125 mg IV), which may not parallel real-world care. Readers should also note that there was a high failure rate among both groups (>50%). While oral medications were not inferior to IV, a majority of patients required hospitalization demonstrating the morbidity associated with COPD. However, the use of oral steroids in the treatment of mild COPD is now a part of many quality improvement campaigns in EDs and hospitals.

Question
Are IV steroids more effective than oral steroids in the treatment of acute COPD exacerbations?

Answer
No, oral steroids are not inferior to IV steroids for patients with COPD exacerbations.

CHAPTER 80: ANTIBIOTICS IN COPD EXACERBATIONS

Antibiotics in Chronic Obstructive Pulmonary Disease Exacerbations. A Meta-Analysis
Saint S, Bent S, Vittinghoff E, Grady D. *JAMA.* 1995;273(12):957–960

BACKGROUND
Chronic obstructive pulmonary disease (COPD) is a common and serious condition, affecting 6% of the US population and killing 120,000 people per year, with an economic impact of $39 billion annually. Prior to this study, antibiotics were routinely administered to patients presenting with COPD exacerbations despite the fact that viral upper respiratory tract infections were the most common cause of such exacerbations. Previous studies examining the effect of routine antibiotics on COPD exacerbations were limited by small sample sizes.

OBJECTIVES
To determine if and to what extent routine administration of antibiotics to patients with COPD exacerbations affects outcomes.

METHODS
Meta-analysis with a priori article inclusion and exclusion criteria of articles from multiple databases published between 1955 and 1994.

Patients
Two hundred and thirty-nine studies were screened, of which nine randomized placebo-controlled trials were included for a total of 1,101 patients in hospital and outpatient settings. Specific patient inclusion and exclusion criteria varied considerably by study.

Intervention Evaluated
Routine administration of antibiotics to patients with COPD exacerbations. Specific antibiotics varied by study.

Outcomes
The effect size of the primary outcome of each study, normalized to the mean and standard deviation in that study, was evaluated. This allowed for comparison of different primary outcomes from each study, including duration of illness and scores on various symptom scales. The change in peak expiratory flow rate (PEFR) was also evaluated.

KEY RESULTS
- An overall effect size of 0.22 was found, favoring the administration of antibiotics by 0.25 standard deviations of the individual outcome that were measured (days of illness, symptom score, etc.).
- Patient who received antibiotics had a PEFR improvement of 10.75 L/min.
- The results were not altered by multiple different weightings of the studies and sensitivity analysis.
- Studies considering only hospitalized patients tended to show greater benefit.

STUDY CONCLUSIONS
Routine administration of antibiotics to patients with COPD exacerbations resulted in small, but statistically significant and clinically significant improvements.

COMMENTARY
This study was designed to more rigorously evaluate the benefit of the already-common practice of routine antibiotic administration for COPD. The strict methodology of the article inclusion and exclusion criteria strengthens the conclusions. Study limitations include the potential for publication bias, lack of adverse event data, and differing antibiotic regimens, which is particularly relevant given that some but not all are known to have immunomodulatory properties and many COPD exacerbations do not have bacterial causes. Despite these limitations, this study provided significant evidence that routine antibiotic administration in COPD exacerbations improves clinical outcomes. More recent studies and guidelines have built on this work by examining other antibiotic choices and identifying subsets of patients most likely to benefit from their administration.

Question
Does routine administration of antibiotics improve clinical outcomes in patients with COPD exacerbations?

Answer
Yes, routine administration of antibiotics for severe exacerbations can decrease illness duration and improve symptom scores.

CHAPTER 81

PULSE-OXIMETRY REPLACES ARTERIAL BLOOD GASES

Impact of Portable Pulse Oximetry on Arterial Blood Gas Test Ordering in an Urban Emergency Department
Kellerman A, Cofer CA, Joseph S, Hackman BB. *Ann Emerg Med.* 1991;20(2): 130–134

BACKGROUND
Prior to this study, arterial blood gas (ABG) testing was routinely performed on patients in the ED to determine whether their oxygenation was adequate. Based on price and frequency ordered they were rated as one of the 10 most costly ED tests. Large bedside pulse oximeters were used in the operating room and intensive care units, and portable battery-powered pulse oximeters were becoming more available. While these provided an alternative measurement of oxygenation, there were no studies demonstrating usability or utility or effect on management in the ED.

OBJECTIVE
To determine whether introduction of a portable pulse oximetry monitor in the ED affected rates of ABG testing.

METHODS
Observational before-and-after study of all ABGs ordered in a single academic ED.

Patients
A total of 20,120 patients visit during a 4-month observation period (9,621 in the 2 months prior to introduction of pulse oximetry and 10,499 in the 2 months after introduction).

Intervention Evaluated
Introduction of a single portable pulse oximeter along with a 5-minute training session on its use. All ABGs ordered in a noncode situation required a pulse oximeter reading be included.

Outcomes
The primary outcome was the number of ABGs performed before and after the introduction of pulse oximetry, along with the indications for ABGs ordered. Secondary outcomes to evaluate safety included unexpected cardiac arrest in the ED, death within 24 hours of admission, and death within 2 days of ED discharge.

KEY RESULTS
- There was a 37% decrease in total ABGs ordered
- There was a 45% decrease in number of repeat ABGs
- Seventy-one percent fewer ABGs were ordered for the purpose of assessing oxygenation only (p-value not reported)
- The number of ABGs indicated by American College of Emergency Physician (ACEP) clinical criteria remained similar before and after the introduction of pulse oximetry (67% vs. 64%)
- No adverse events were recorded before or after the intervention

STUDY CONCLUSIONS
Introduction of pulse oximetry reduced ABG ordering by 37%, mostly due to decreased testing to detect abnormalities of oxygenation. No major adverse events occurred before or after the intervention.

COMMENTARY
This study provided evidence supporting the concept that pulse oximetry can be used to replace the ABG analysis that had previously been performed to evaluate oxygenation. While 71% fewer ABGs were ordered to assess oxygenation only, it is not reported what percentage of the total decrease can be attributed to this subset. It is possible that some of the decrease is attributable to unrelated causes, such as house staff gaining more clinical experience and therefore relying less on ancillary testing. Although no adverse events were reported, this may represent a failure to capture minor events or major events of a very low baseline frequency, and does not conclusively prove the absence of harm. Overall, this study demonstrates a significantly decreased rate of ABG testing and suggests that it was at least partially related to substituting pulse oximetry to detect abnormalities of oxygenation only. In its broader historical context, this study led to common use of noninvasive oxygenation monitoring and created the conceptual framework for noninvasive monitoring of ventilation, which is becoming increasingly prevalent.

Question
Has the use of portable pulse oximetry decreased arterial blood gas (ABG) testing?

Answer
Yes, the introduction of noninvasive oxygenation monitoring has decreased ABG testing.

SECTION 14
TOXICOLOGY

Sabrina J. Poon ■ Fan Yang ■ Spencer Greene ■ Silpa Gadiraju

82. Fomepizole in Ethylene Glycol Poisoning
83. Hyperbaric Oxygen in Carbon Monoxide Poisoning
84. The Rumack–Matthew Nomogram: Acetaminophen Poisoning and Toxicity
85. NAC in Acetaminophen Overdose
86. Cyanide Poisoning and Hydroxocobalamin
87. Digitalis Toxicity and Digoxin Immune Fab
88. Crofab in Snakebites

CHAPTER 82: FOMEPIZOLE IN ETHYLENE GLYCOL POISONING

Fomepizole for the Treatment of Ethylene Glycol Poisoning
Brent J, McMartin K, Phillips S, et al. *N Engl J Med.* 1999;340(11):832–838

BACKGROUND
Ethylene glycol poisoning causes significant morbidity, including renal failure, damage to the central nervous system, and cardiovascular instability. Prior to this study the standard treatment of ethylene glycol poisoning included high-dose ethanol as a means of inhibiting the conversion of ethylene glycol into its toxic metabolites through alcohol dehydrogenase. Ethanol has concerning side effects including intoxication, hepatotoxicity, and hypoglycemia as well as a widely variable metabolism. Fomepizole is an inhibitor of alcohol dehydrogenase that, at the time of this study, was theorized to have similar clinical benefit as high-dose alcohol in the treatment of ethylene glycol poisoning without the toxic side effects.

OBJECTIVES
To determine the efficacy of fomepizole in the treatment of ethylene glycol poisoning.

METHODS
Prospective, open, multicenter study between 1995 and 1997.

Participants
19 patients >12 years old who met one of three sets of criteria were included: (1) plasma ethylene glycol concentration ≥20 mg/dL, (2) suspected ingestion and at least three of four specific laboratory findings (arterial pH <7.3, serum bicarbonate <20 mmol/L, serum osmolar gap >10 mOsm/L, and oxaluria), or (3) suspected ingestion within 1 hour and a serum osmolar gap >10 mOsm/L.

Intervention Evaluated
IV fomepizole given over at least 2 days, with more doses given until the plasma ethylene glycol concentration was <20 mg/dL. Patients also underwent hemodialysis if they met specific criteria including severe metabolic acidosis, high creatinine, or high initial ethylene glycol concentration.

Outcomes
The primary outcome was renal injury as defined by elevated creatinine. Secondary outcomes included additional production of ethylene glycol metabolites as defined by increases in plasma glycolate concentration or urinary oxalate excretion, as well as cranial neuropathies.

KEY RESULTS
- Nine out of 19 patients developed renal injury, which resolved in six patients. Ten patients did not develop renal injury.
- When compared with the patients who did not develop renal failure, those that did tended to present later (15.1 vs. 9.6 hours), and at the time of presentation had abnormal renal function (creatinine 2.2 vs. 0.9), higher glycolate levels (159 vs. 28.1), more severe acidosis (arterial pH 7.14 vs. 7.34), and lower bicarbonate (6.8 vs. 17.8). All of the patients who did not develop renal injury had a normal creatinine at presentation and a plasma glycolate concentration <76.8 mg/dL.
- Plasma glycolate concentrations and urinary oxalate excretion decreased in all patients.
- None of the patients developed a cranial neuropathy.

STUDY CONCLUSIONS
When administered early, fomepizole prevents renal injury in patients with ethylene glycol poisoning. The investigators found that acidosis improved as plasma glycolate concentration decreased.

COMMENTARY
Given the potentially devastating effects of ethylene glycol poisoning, this study provided evidence that in comparison to ethanol, fomepizole is an effective alternative with a low side effect profile and more predictable pharmacokinetics. This pivotal study prospectively validated the use of fomepizole in a series of patients with ethylene glycol poisoning, and most importantly, proved its efficacy in preventing renal injury. Subsequently, this study led to the same group publishing another trial that validated the use of fomepizole for treating methanol poisoning, which has also become the standard of care. Although fomepizole is the official antidote for ethylene glycol poisoning as recommended by the American Academy of Clinical Toxicology, if unavailable, ethanol could be used as an alternative, albeit an unproven one with significant safety concerns. Also important to consider is the role of hemodialysis, which most of the patients in this study underwent. Subsequent papers have suggested that fomepizole alone without hemodialysis is sufficient to prevent renal injury; however, deciding whether or not to pursue hemodialysis should be made in conjunction with the appropriate consultants.

Question
Is fomepizole an effective treatment for ethylene glycol poisoning?

Answer
Yes, fomepizole decreases severe renal injury when used in patients with a suspected ingestion, metabolic acidosis, or an osmolar gap of unknown etiology.

CHAPTER 83

HYPERBARIC OXYGEN IN CARBON MONOXIDE POISONING

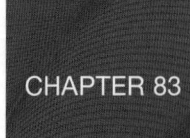

Hyperbaric Oxygen for Acute Carbon Monoxide Poisoning
Weaver LK, Hopkins RO, Chan KJ, et al. *N Engl J Med.* 2002;347(14):1057–1067

BACKGROUND
Carbon monoxide (CO) poisoning was responsible for 40,000 ED visits around the time of this study with cognitive impairment resulting in up to a quarter of patients who had lost consciousness or had carboxyhemoglobin levels >25%. While some studies reported superior outcomes in patients treated with hyperbaric oxygen (HBO), at the time of this study the evidence around its efficacy was conflicting in comparison to 100% normobaric oxygen. As HBO is costly and can present a transport issue to select HBO centers, it was not clear that the evidence supported this therapy.

OBJECTIVES
To determine the effect of HBO on cognitive sequelae (changes in memory, attention, and effect) in patients with CO poisoning.

METHODS
Prospective, multicenter, double-blind, randomized trial conducted at a single referral center from 1992 to 1999.

Participants
152 patients, >16 years old, with symptomatic acute CO poisoning, as defined by exposure to CO within 24 hours of presentation in conjunction with prespecified symptoms. Select exclusion criteria: >24 hours since their exposure to CO, moribund, or pregnant.

Intervention Evaluated
Three chamber sessions within a 24-hour period consisting of either three hyperbaric oxygen treatments or one normobaric oxygen treatment plus two sessions of exposure to room air.

Outcomes
The primary outcome was cognitive sequelae 6 weeks after CO poisoning as measured by neuropsychological tests. Secondary outcomes included test scores at various time intervals after CO poisoning, a selfreport questionnaire of symptoms at 6 weeks, scores on three validated scales, and results of a neurologic examination after the third chamber session.

KEY RESULTS
- Cognitive sequelae at 6 weeks were significantly less frequent in the HBO group than in the normobaric/room air group (25% vs. 46.1%).
- Cognitive sequelae were significantly less frequent in the HBO group at 6 months (21.1% vs. 38.2%) and 12 months (18.4% vs. 32.9%).
- At 6 weeks, patients in the HBO group reported fewer difficulties with memory, but an insignificant difference in attention or concentration ($p = 0.17$).
- Adverse events of treatment included anxiety, tympanic membrane rupture, cough, and difficulty equalizing middle-ear pressure.

STUDY CONCLUSIONS
Three HBO treatments within 24 hours reduce the risk of cognitive sequelae 6 weeks and 12 months after CO poisoning. HBO is recommended for patients with acute CO poisoning.

COMMENTARY
The existence of hyperbaric oxygen treatment centers has increased greatly over the last century, and along with it the list of indications for its use, some with conflicting evidence such as CO poisoning. The methodology of this paper is impressive in its blinded and randomized nature, as well as its intention-to-treat analysis, especially since significantly more patients failed to complete treatment in the HBO group (18.4% vs. 3.9%). Also impressive is the primary outcome of cognitive sequelae, since it is a meaningful longitudinal patient outcome. However, the effects of HBO may be overstated due to the intervention of three hyperbaric sessions vs. one normobaric session, as this does not exclude the possibility that two extra treatments alone, and not the modality of treatment, cause the difference in outcome. In addition, the HBO group had less severe cerebellar dysfunction than the other group (15% vs. 4%), though the conclusion was found to hold after the authors adjusted for baseline differences. A 2011 Cochrane review concluded that the existing trials, including this one, are insufficient in providing evidence for the role of HBO in reducing adverse neurologic outcomes from CO poisoning. Despite the review, this trial has made CO poisoning the most common reason for acute HBO, and has created a national change in the standard of care for severe CO poisonings in which transfer for HBO has become expected and mentioned as "should be considered" in clinical practice guidelines.

Question
Does hyperbaric oxygen therapy improve outcomes in carbon monoxide poisoning?

Answer
Yes, hyperbaric oxygen treatment decreases delayed neuropsychological symptoms in severe carbon monoxide exposures.

CHAPTER 84

THE RUMACK–MATTHEW NOMOGRAM: ACETAMINOPHEN POISONING AND TOXICITY

Acetaminophen Poisoning and Toxicity
Rumack BH, Matthew H. *Pediatrics.* 1975;55(6):871–876

BACKGROUND
Acetaminophen toxicity is insidious, leading to varied outcomes ranging from spontaneous recovery to fulminant hepatic failure. In 1975, Rumack and Matthew performed the first and to date largest observation study investigating the prognostic value of serum acetaminophen levels over time in predicting hepatotoxicity in untreated overdoses. Previous works had established that if at 12 hours postingestion acetaminophen levels were <50 mcg/mL, there was a very low likelihood of hepatic injury. This study was addressing missing information in prognosis as N-acetylcysteine (NAC) had not yet been discovered at the time of this study.

OBJECTIVE
To correlate serum acetaminophen levels over time with outcomes of hepatotoxicity in untreated cases of acetaminophen intoxication.

METHODS
Observational study by Rumack and Matthew, combined with observational data by previous investigators performed at two study centers in the early 1970s, although the authors did not provide dates of enrollment.

Participants
64 Acetaminophen overdose cases.

Intervention Evaluated
Documented acetaminophen and aspartate transaminase (AST) levels over time combined with known 12 hour postingestion level.

Outcomes
AST >1,000 during hospitalization was used as a surrogate for possible hepatic injury.

KEY RESULTS
- No hepatotoxicity was observed in patients with acetaminophen levels <200 at four hours after ingestion and <50 at 12 hours post ingestion.
- Nomogram was plotted out to 16 hours, which corresponds to four acetaminophen half-lives.
- Nomogram only applies to acute single-dose ingestion with clear time of ingestion.

Chapter 84 ■ The Rumack–Matthew Nomogram: Acetaminophen Poisoning and Toxicity

COMMENTARY

The Rumack–Matthew nomogram was published around the time that NAC was discovered to be an effective treatment of acetaminophen toxicity. The nomogram provided the only evidence-based algorithm evaluating the risk of hepatotoxicity in untreated patients, and consequently answered the critical question of which patients required treatment for acetaminophen overdose. It is a unique study that will never be repeated given the absence of clinical equipoise for withholding NAC treatment.

These data informed the U.S. Food and Drug Administration modification that lowered the threshold for hepatotoxicity by 25% as a safety margin, which resulted in to the "150" at four-hour rule currently used in emergency medicine. The safety of withholding treatment for patients who have acetaminophen levels below the nomogram line has been repeatedly validated and is now the standard of care. The major caveat of this study and the nomogram is the reliance on ingestion time, which can often be impossible to determine. As such, ingestions associated with suicide attempts, staggered ingestions, ingestion of extended-release formulas, chronic intoxication, and ingestions along with GI motility-slowing agents should preclude the use of nomogram. In clinical practice, the nomogram cannot be used in a minority of patients (up to 44% in one study), for whom NAC therapy should be initiated empirically.

Question

Is N-acetylcysteine therapy indicated in all patients with acetaminophen overdose?

Answer

No, therapy is indicated if the patient's acetaminophen level is above 150 mcg/mL at 4 hours postingestion, or above the nomogram treatment line at any subsequent point. If a patient's acetaminophen level at 4 hours or later is below the nomogram threshold and the history of ingestion is reliable, it is reasonable to discharge the patient.

CHAPTER 85
NAC IN ACETAMINOPHEN OVERDOSE

Efficacy of Oral N-acetylcysteine in the Treatment of Acetaminophen Overdose
Smilkstein MJ, Knapp GL, Kulig KW, Rumack BH. *N Engl J Med.* 1988;319(24):1557–1562

BACKGROUND
Acetaminophen toxicity is the most common drug toxicity leading to hepatic failure. In 1975, Rumack and Matthew published the first nomogram of plasma acetaminophen level as it pertained to hepatic toxicity at the same time that N-acetylcysteine (NAC) was developed as a possible antidote. A decade later, there was increasing interest in the true efficacy of NAC and appropriate timing of administration.

OBJECTIVES
To determine the efficacy of oral NAC in preventing acetaminophen-induced hepatotoxicity as it related to both the initial plasma acetaminophen concentration and the delay before treatment initiation.

METHODS
National, prospective, open, multicenter study between September 1976 and February 1985.

Patients
2,540 patients with a measured plasma acetaminophen concentration between 4 and 24 hours after ingestion above 150 mcg/mL at 4 hours, or an estimated ingestion of 7.5 g in an adult or 140 mg/kg in a child. 2,023 of these patients had acetaminophen levels above the study nomogram line.

Intervention Evaluated
A loading dose of NAC, followed 4 hours later by the first of 17 doses of NAC, all administered orally or via a gastric or enteral tube.

Outcomes
The primary outcome was hepatotoxicity (AST or ALT >1,000 International Unit/L) as it related to (1) patients treated with NAC within 10 hours and between 10 and 24 hours after ingestion in both probable-risk and high-risk subgroups, (2) initial plasma acetaminophen concentrations in patients who were treated with NAC within 8 hours of ingestion, and (3) delay in treatment by 4-hour increments.

KEY RESULTS
- Hepatotoxicity developed in significantly fewer patients treated within 10 hours vs. those treated between 10 and 24 hours after ingestion in both the probable-risk subgroup (6.1% vs. 26.4%) and the high-risk subgroup (8.3% vs. 34.4%).
- Hepatotoxicity was uncommon in all patients who were treated within 8 hours of ingestion, regardless of initial plasma acetaminophen level.
- There was no difference in ALT or AST levels for patients treated within the first 8 hours after ingestion, but beyond 8 hours increasing liver damage was measured.

STUDY CONCLUSIONS
The risk of hepatotoxicity is minimal when NAC treatment is initiated within 8 hours of acetaminophen ingestion, regardless of initial serum acetaminophen concentration.

COMMENTARY
This study filled an important knowledge gap regarding the critical time window for NAC treatment—within 8 hours of ingestion was universally successful. This generous time window should not result in a treatment delay, but rather provide the physician with adequate time to obtain and plot the acetaminophen level on the nomogram and determine whether to administer NAC. As part of the trial, the U.S. Food and Drug Administration also required that a safety line intersecting 150 mcg/mL at 4 hours be added to the initial nomogram, which is the nomogram that is in use today. As proven in this and other research since, NAC is a safe drug with marked therapeutic benefits. The nomogram does, however, have several limitations, including that it is only useful after a single acute ingestion, and that an accurate timeline can be difficult to obtain in some cases. As a result NAC therapy can be liberally initiated in patients with suspected acetaminophen toxicity.

Question
How quickly must NAC be administered in acetaminophen ingestions?

Answer
If NAC is given within the first 8 hours after acetaminophen ingestion, the risk of hepatotoxicity is virtually eliminated.

CHAPTER 86
CYANIDE POISONING AND HYDROXOCOBALAMIN

Prospective Study of Hydroxocobalamin for Acute Cyanide Poisoning in Smoke Inhalation
Borron SW, Baud FJ, Barriot P, Imbert M, Bismuth C. *Ann Emerg Med.* 2007; 49(6):794–801

BACKGROUND
Cyanide poisoning has long been recognized as a significant health hazard from fire smoke inhalation, with untreated mortality exceeding 50%. The cyanide that is produced from the combustion of nitrogen- and carbon-containing substances (i.e., foam, plastics, nylon, wool) causes a cellular hypoxia that leads to altered mental status, cardiovascular instability, and a significant metabolic acidosis. While a cyanide antidote kit consisting of amyl nitrite, sodium nitrite, and sodium thiosulfate was found to reduce the morbidity and mortality of cyanide toxicity, it often went unused because of the risk of methemoglobinemia from concurrent smoke inhalation. Hydroxocobalamin, a vitamin B12 precursor, has been licensed for use in France since 1996. It received FDA approval in 2006 for the treatment of acute cyanide toxicity despite a paucity of prospective evaluation.

OBJECTIVES
To determine if empiric, prehospital administration of hydroxocobalamin could safely and effectively treat patients with acute cyanide toxicity following smoke inhalation.

METHODS
Prospective, observational case series of patients treated for smoke inhalation by the Paris Fire Brigade between 1987 and 1994.

Patients
69 patients, >15 years old, with evidence of smoke inhalation and abnormal neurologic status defined as disturbances of consciousness, slowed ideation, agitation, or mental confusion. Select exclusion criteria: Obviously gravid women and patients with burns on the neck and face or with second-degree burns >20% body surface area.

Intervention Evaluated
Treatment with hydroxocobalamin infused over 15 to 30 minutes was begun after an initial blood draw. Additional doses up to a maximum of 15 g could be administered at the discretion of the treating physician for incomplete hemodynamic or neurologic response.

Outcomes
The primary outcome was survival. Secondary outcomes included amelioration of neurologic signs, hemodynamic characteristics (heart rate, blood pressure), neuropsychiatric sequelae, and adverse events following treatment with hydroxocobalamin.

KEY RESULTS
- 67% (28/42) of patients treated with hydroxocobalamin survived.
- 51% (21/41) of patients with neurologic impairment improved and had no sequelae after treatment with hydroxocobalamin.
- 27.5% (19/69) of patients treated with hydroxocobalamin experienced one or more adverse events such as chromaturia, skin erythema, or hypertension. No allergic reactions were noted.

STUDY CONCLUSIONS
Empiric administration of hydroxocobalamin improved survival and neurologic recovery of patient suffering from cyanide toxicity due to smoke inhalation. Intravenous hydroxocobalamin is associated with a low rate of adverse events with minor clinical significance.

COMMENTARY
This study is the largest to evaluate the efficacy of hydroxocobalamin for the treatment of cyanide toxicity in the setting of smoke inhalation, and the results are certainly encouraging. There were no significant adverse effects reported, though other studies have described allergic reactions requiring treatment with corticosteroids, interference on laboratory tests, and a variety of symptoms, including chest pain, nausea, dysphagia, and pruritus. What this study does not do, however, is compare the efficacy of hydroxocobalamin to sodium thiosulfate, which to date has not been studied. It should also be noted that in this study it was physicians who treated the patients in the prehospital environment, which is different from how out-of-hospital medicine is practiced in the United States. The significance of this difference is uncertain, but it is possible French prehospital providers are better able to diagnose and treat toxicity from cyanide and other fire gases than nonphysician providers in the United States. The vast majority of US EMS systems now carry hydroxocobalamin for empiric prehospital treatment of obtunded or unstable patients exposed to massive smoke inhalation.

Question
Can hydroxocobalamin safely and effectively treat patients with acute cyanide toxicity following smoke inhalation?

Answer
Yes, empiric administration of hydroxocobalamin appears to reduce mortality in acute cyanide poisoning.

CHAPTER 87
DIGITALIS TOXICITY AND DIGOXIN IMMUNE FAB

Treatment of 150 Cases of Life-Threatening Digitalis Intoxication With Digoxin-specific Fab Antibody Fragments: Final Report of a Multicenter Study
Antman EM, Wenger TL, Butler VP Jr, Haber E, Smith TW. *Circulation.* 1990; 81(6):1744–1752

BACKGROUND
The effects of digitalis toxicity can be life-threatening, and include lethal arrhythmias such as AV block and ventricular tachycardia. Although the use of digoxin-specific antibody (Fab) fragments to treat digoxin toxicity was first described in 1976, at the time of this study Fab had not been tested across a broad set of patients, and adequate safety information for drug approval had not yet been obtained. Today, the antidote is marketed under the trade names DigiFab and Digibind.

OBJECTIVES
To determine the ability of Fab fragments to reverse the toxic effects of digitalis, and to assess its safety.

METHODS
Open-label multicenter clinical trial conducted in 21 centers between 1974 and 1986.

Participants
150 patients with known digitalis exposure and actual or potentially life-threatening cardiac rhythm disturbances and/or hyperkalemia actually or likely to be refractory to conventional therapies. Of the patients, 50% were on long-term digitalis therapy, 10% had an accidental overdose, and 39% had overdosed with suicidal intent.

Intervention Evaluated
A dose of Fab fragments based on the amount of digoxin or digitoxin calculated to be in the patient's body, either estimated from the medical history or determined by serum concentration.

Outcomes
The primary outcomes were efficacy of Fab fragments in reversing the toxic effects of digitalis and adverse drug events. The secondary outcomes were the pharmacokinetics and pharmacodynamics of Fab and its antigenicity in humans.

KEY RESULTS
- The clinical response to Fab was obtained in 148 patients: 80% (119) resolved all signs and symptoms of digitalis toxicity, 10% (14) improved, and 10% (15) had no response.
- Time course data was obtained for 80 of the patients with complete resolution of symptoms: The average time to initial response was 19 minutes (0 to 60 minutes), and the average time to complete response was 88 minutes (30 to 360 minutes).
- 14/150 patients had adverse events possibly or probably caused by Fab including hypokalemia, exacerbations of congestive heart failure, mild hypotensive episodes, nausea, and transient apnea in a neonate.
- The serum concentration of pharmacologically active digoxin or digitoxin was nearly 0 within 1 to 2 minutes of Fab treatment.

STUDY CONCLUSIONS
In patients who are treated for digitalis toxicity with Fab fragments, a response to treatment can be expected in at least 90% of patients with advanced and/or life-threatening toxicity.

COMMENTARY
The treatment for digoxin toxicity before the advent of Fab fragments was limited to supportive care. Although this was an open-label study in which the lack of blinding or an active control could mean that concomitant supportive therapy may have yielded some of the efficacy, this research provided convincing evidence supporting the effectiveness of Fab fragments as first-line therapy in digoxin toxicity. The vast majority of patients demonstrated clinical improvement and free serum digoxin was nearly eliminated by treatment. It is important to note that as fewer and fewer outpatients are on chronic digoxin therapy for atrial fibrillation, the antidote may have limited applicability. Regardless, the development and use of this antidote is broadly supported by toxicologists for any suspected patient with digoxin overdose with cardiovascular instability.

Question
Do Fab fragments improve outcomes in patients with digoxin toxicity?

Answer
Yes, Fab treatment is recommended for severely symptomatic or life-threatening cases of digoxin toxicity, including patients with arrhythmias, renal dysfunction, or hyperkalemia.

CHAPTER 88 CROFAB IN SNAKEBITES

A Randomized Multicenter Trial of Crotalinae Polyvalent Immune Fab (Ovine) Antivenom for the Treatment for Crotaline Snakebite in the United States
Dart RC, Seifert SA, Boyer LV, et al. *Arch Intern Med.* 2001;161(16):2030–2036

BACKGROUND
Out of the several thousand snakebite victims every year in the United States, approximately six die and an additional 15% to 40% suffer long-term complications of envenomation from minor limb disfiguration to coagulopathic and neurologic dysfunction. The previously available horse serum antivenom was effective against venomous Crotalidae bites but had several potential adverse effects such as acute hypersensitivity reactions (urticaria, hypotension, anaphylaxis) and delayed hypersensitivity reactions (serum sickness). A new ovine antivenom, Crotalinae polyvalent immune Fab (Fab AV) was shown to be safe and effective in a prospective open-label pilot trial involving 11 patients; however, local recurrence of limb swelling was observed in several patients, prompting this first randomized trial of antivenin in the United States.

OBJECTIVES
To compare the safety and efficacy of two dosing regimens of Crotalinae polyvalent immune Fab (Fab AV).

METHODS
Prospective, randomized, open-label comparative trial of two dosing regimens of Fab AV performed at seven sites in six US states between 1994 and 1996. A validated severity score was used to assess patient severity.

Participants
Thirty-one patients, >10 years old, presenting within 6 hours of minimal or moderate envenomation by a Crotalinae snake and with progression of the envenomation syndrome. Select exclusion criteria: Patients with severe venom poisoning or bite by a copperhead snake.

Interventions
First a dose was administered to obtain initial control. Subsequently, patients were randomized into two groups: (1) A scheduled group which received Fab AV every 6 hours for 18 hours, and (2) a PRN group which could receive two vial increments as needed if there was continued progression of coagulopathy, local, or systemic effects.

Outcomes
The primary outcome was initial control of the envenomation syndrome measured using the snakebite severity score. Secondary outcomes included safety measurements (acute and delayed hypersensitivity reactions), local or coagulopathic recurrence and time to reconstitute the antivenom.

KEY RESULTS
- Initial control of the envenomation syndrome was achieved in all patients.
- Twenty-three percent developed an acute reaction during Fab AV infusion with the same number (23%) developing serum sickness noted at 14-day follow-up.
- The mean severity score of the 31 patients decreased from 4.35 to 2.39 points with the components of the severity score involving the coagulation system, central nervous system, cardiovascular system, and gastrointestinal tract all decreased throughout the evaluation period.
- There was no statistical difference between the scheduled and PRN groups. However, 50% (8) of patients in the PRN group required additional doses for recurrence of wound progression during the first 12 hours ($p = 0.002$). A return of coagulation abnormalities was noted in many patients who exhibited a coagulopathy at presentation.

STUDY CONCLUSIONS
Fab AV effectively terminated venom effects in both the scheduled and PRN groups. As unplanned additional doses of Fab AV were common in the PRN group, the treatment regimen may require more than one initial dose.

COMMENTARY
Due to the perceived risks associated with the previously available antivenom ACP, and lack of any prospective data in the United States, many physicians delayed giving treatment, or gave too small a dose of antivenin. In this first prospective randomized trial of antivenom in the United States, the newer antivenin Fab AV demonstrated fewer adverse reactions and termination of local recurrent with repeated doses in comparison to ACP. Limitations of this study include its open-label design with potential investigator bias, the lack of an untreated control group, and that severe envenomation patients were excluded from the study as were those inflicted by copperhead bites. Also five out of six patients who developed serum sickness were found to have received antivenin with excess Fc fragments due to flaws in the manufacturing process, making the true rate of serum sickness difficult to gauge and highlighting the potential for flaws in manufacturing.

The PRN arm of this study demonstrated the need for adequate antivenin should be available for potential additional doses to treat recurrence after initial control.

Question
Does polyvalent immune Fab AV reduce harm from snakebites?

Answer
Yes, Fab AV can be used safely and effectively to control envenomation syndrome in Crotalinae snake bites.

SECTION 15
TRAUMA

Andrew J. Eyre ■ Eva Tovar Hirashima ■ David Beversluis

89. Laparotomy in Abdominal Gunshot Wounds
90. Permissive Hypotension in Trauma
91. Level One Trauma Centers
92. CT vs. X-Ray in Traumatic Cervical Spine Injury
93. The NEXUS Criteria and the Canadian C-Spine Rules
94. New Orleans Criteria and the Canadian Head CT Rules
95. ED Thoracotomies
96. Pediatric Head Trauma

CHAPTER 89
LAPAROTOMY IN ABDOMINAL GUNSHOT WOUNDS

Selective Nonoperative Management in 1,856 Patients with Abdominal Gunshot Wounds: Should Routine Laparotomy Still be the Standard of Care?
Velmahos GC, Demetriades D, Toutouzas KG, et al. *Ann Surg.* 2001;234(3):395–402

BACKGROUND
Abdominal gunshot wounds (GSWs) are a frequent and high-mortality injury seen in many EDs. Traditional practice in most trauma centers for these injuries has been routine laparotomy due to a perceived high incidence of significant intra-abdominal injury, the supposed harmless nature of a laparotomy, and the unreliability of physical examination. Prior to this study, selective nonoperative management in patients with blunt trauma and penetrating stab wounds had been shown to be safe and cost effective; however, no evidence existed to support this approach in GSW patients.

OBJECTIVES
To describe the experience of 8 years of a selective nonoperative management protocol in abdominal GSW patients and to evaluate its effect on safety, cost, efficiency, and length of stay.

METHODS
Retrospective observational study conducted in a single Level I trauma center in the US between 1993 and 2000.

Participants
1,856 patients with anterior and posterior abdominal GSWs. Select exclusion criteria: Patients with an obviously superficial GSW or who underwent ED thoracotomy and died shortly after admission.

Interventions
A policy of selective nonoperative management in anterior and posterior abdominal GSW patients who did not have peritonitis, were stable and had a reliable abdominal examination.

Outcomes
Primary outcome was the number of patients selected for nonoperative management and the subset of these requiring delayed laparotomy, as well as the percentage who underwent initial laparotomy and the subset of these who underwent unnecessary laparotomy. Secondary outcomes were length and cost of hospital stay.

KEY RESULTS
- 42% (792) underwent selective nonoperative management; 4% (80) required delayed laparotomy, and 57 of these discovered injury that required repair. 38% (712) were discharged without surgery.
- 9% (163) of all patients were deemed to have undergone unnecessary surgery; if all patients had undergone initial routine laparotomy 47% would have undergone unnecessary surgery.
- 3,560 hospital days and $9.5 million were saved over the study period by use of this approach compared to a hypothetical routine laparotomy policy in the same patients.

STUDY CONCLUSIONS
Selective nonoperative management for abdominal GSWs is a safe management strategy at trauma centers with an in-house trauma team and significantly reduces unnecessary laparotomies as well as the cost of care.

COMMENTARY
The previous standard of care had been for routine laparotomy for almost all abdominal GSWs; this study was designed to rebut this traditional approach given the high negative laparotomy rate and long-term complications associated with abdominal surgery. This retrospective study does not allow for a direct comparison between the nonoperative and routine management cohorts, the latter being a much sicker population by definition. Rather, they report adjusted outcomes to show that over 40% of their cohort was eligible for a nonoperative approach and did very well, with the majority able to be discharged without complications or need for a laparotomy. These findings need to be applied with some caution as not all centers have the ability to perform serial abdominal examinations in house or ready access to surgical alternatives such as interventional radiology to manage potential intra-abdominal injuries. Also, the author's regression analyses does not identify any significant predictors of a successful nonoperative outcome, as such selecting patients for this approach is challenging. These results prompted many trauma centers to adopt this approach and set the stage for further research into the use of other nonoperative interventions including angiographic embolization.

Question
Are there patients with abdominal gunshot wounds who can be managed nonoperatively?

Answer
Yes, stable patients with a reliable examination and without peritonitis can be safely managed nonoperatively if they undergo serial abdominal examinations.

CHAPTER 90: PERMISSIVE HYPOTENSION IN TRAUMA

Immediate vs. Delayed Fluid Resuscitation for Hypotensive Patients with Penetrating Torso Injuries
Bickell WH, Wall MJ Jr, Pepe PE, et al. *NEJM*. 1994;331(17):1105–1109

BACKGROUND
Aggressive isotonic fluid administration was a standard in trauma resuscitation for many years; however, increasing evidence in the early 1990s suggested a restrictive strategy might be beneficial. It was postulated that aggressive administration of fluids can disrupt thrombus formation and increase bleeding. This study was an early attempt to compare a delayed vs. standard approach in trauma patients and assess for mortality benefit.

OBJECTIVES
To determine whether hypotensive penetrating trauma patients who have fluid resuscitation delayed until the time of operative intervention have improved survival compared to patient receiving standard fluid resuscitation.

METHODS
Prospective trial with even–odd day assignments to two treatment arms in a Houston area EMS system and primary trauma hospital between 1989 and 1992.

Participants
598 of 1,069 patients were enrolled. Inclusion criteria: Age ≥16 years, gunshot or stab wound to the torso, initial on-scene systolic blood pressure <90. Select exclusion criteria: Pregnant, death, fatal gunshot wound to head, or minor injuries not requiring operative intervention. 309 were in the immediate-resuscitation group and 289 were in the delayed-resuscitation group.

Interventions
Patients were either given immediate standard intravenous fluid (IVF) resuscitation by paramedics and the trauma team or fluid resuscitation was delayed until arrival in the operating room.

Outcomes
The primary outcome was survival to hospital discharge. The secondary outcomes were amount of intraoperative hemorrhage, length of hospitalization, and frequency of postoperative complications including: Acute Respiratory Distress Syndrome (ARDS), sepsis syndrome, acute renal failure, coagulopathy, wound infection, and pneumonia.

KEY RESULTS
- There was no statistically significant difference in death prior to arrival to the operating room between the two groups (13% in the immediate-resuscitation group vs. 10% in the delayed-resuscitation group).
- Mean prehospital IVF in the immediate-resuscitation group was 870 mL compared to 92 mL in the delayed-resuscitation group; in-hospital mean volume was 1,608 mL and 283 mL in each group, respectively. There was no significant difference in IVF or blood products administered during surgery.
- Survival was significantly higher in the delayed group compared to the immediate group (70% vs. 62%).
- The immediate-resuscitation group had significantly longer hospital length of stay, but no difference in intensive care unit length of stay.

STUDY CONCLUSIONS
IVF resuscitation of hypotensive penetrating trauma patients with crystalloid should be delayed until the time of surgical control of bleeding to avoid detrimental effects including decreased survival to hospital discharge.

COMMENTARY
Traditional dogma had long been to aggressively give IVF for resuscitation of hypotensive trauma patients. Evidence had begun to accumulate during the prior several decades to support a fluid-restrictive approach. This study was the first to utilize a randomized design combined with a meaningful endpoint (survival to hospital discharge) to show a statistically significant benefit to permissive hypotension. The successful application of these findings requires coordination with the prehospital setting, which the authors carefully coordinate with local EMS to ensure that a restrictive approach actually indicates less IVF. This early data on mortality and associated complications is consistent with subsequent studies that have consistently shown the benefits of restricting crystalloid resuscitation in trauma patients in favor of blood products, a clinical practice that is increasingly reflected in guidelines.

Question
Does fluid resuscitation impact outcomes in hypotensive penetrating trauma victims?

Answer
Yes, patients have improved survival with restrictive and delayed crystalloid resuscitation.

CHAPTER 91
LEVEL ONE TRAUMA CENTERS

A National Evaluation of the Effect of Trauma-center Care on Mortality
MacKenzie EJ, Rivara FP, Jurkovich GJ, et al. *N Engl J Med.* 2006;354(4):366–378

BACKGROUND
As emergency care became more recognized nationally and trauma care algorithms developed, the American College of Surgeons led efforts to regionalize and certify trauma centers to ensure timely trauma care across the United States. This stratification of care was rational but lacked evidence showing a clear mortality benefit. Studies that had been done were complicated by methodologic flaws such as referral bias.

OBJECTIVES
To evaluate the effect of care at a Level I trauma center compared to a nontrauma center on in-hospital and 1-year mortality.

METHODS
A prospective, multicenter observational trial conducted at 18 Level I trauma centers and 51 large nontrauma centers in the United States between 2001 and 2002.

Participants
5,191 trauma patients, 18 to 84 years old, treated for moderate-to-severe injury. Select exclusion criteria: Patients who died within 30 minutes of arrival, delayed treatment for >24 hours from injury, >65 years old with primary diagnosis of hip fracture, or major burns.

Interventions
The mortality associated with care at a Level I trauma center as compared to similar nontrauma centers. Statistical analysis utilized propensity matching based on Abbreviated Injury Scales and comorbidity scales were conducted to adjust for differences between patients from trauma and nontrauma centers due to referral bias.

Outcomes
Primary outcomes were death in the hospital and at 30, 90, and 365 days after injury.

KEY RESULTS
- Patients treated in nontrauma centers were older, had greater comorbidities, and were more likely to be female, non-Hispanic white, insured, and have less severe injuries. After propensity matching these baseline characteristics were similar between groups.
- After adjustment, 1-year mortality in trauma center patients was lower than nontrauma center patients (10.4% vs. 13.8%).
- The greatest benefit associated with trauma centers (trending result) was noted for younger patients and patients with higher injury severity.

STUDY CONCLUSIONS
The overall risk of death is significantly lower when care is provided in a trauma center compared to when provided in a nontrauma center.

COMMENTARY
Over the last two decades there has been a general trend toward regionalization of trauma care as well as several other acute medical services including cardiac and neurologic care. Despite this transition, there was little data supporting the benefits of transferring trauma patients directly to a high-level trauma center. This study, and several other similar studies around the same time, provided some of the first robust evidence that regionalized trauma centers improve patient outcomes. The authors overcome the effect of referral bias, which had prevented prior analysis, through propensity matching and are, therefore, able to make direct comparisons between trauma and nontrauma hospitals in this analysis. With these findings available there has since been an even greater expansion and reinforcement of regionalized specialty trauma care.

Question
Does transfer to a Level 1 trauma center from a nontrauma center improve patient outcomes?

Answer
Yes, patients treated at a trauma center, particularly those who are younger and with a higher injury severity, have significantly lower mortality.

CHAPTER 92
CT VS. X-RAY IN TRAUMATIC CERVICAL SPINE INJURY

Prospective Comparison of Admission Computed Tomographic Scan and Plain Films of the Upper Cervical Spine in Trauma Patients with Altered Mental Status
Schenarts PJ, Diaz J, Kaiser C, et al. *J Trauma*. 2001;51(4):663–668

BACKGROUND
Cervical spine injuries are common in blunt trauma and may result in neurologic deterioration if diagnosis is delayed. Prior to the advent of widely accessible computed tomography (CT) in the 1990s the standard of care had been cervical radiography (plain films) for the diagnosis of traumatic injury when patients had unreliable examinations secondary to altered mental status (AMS). In 1998, the Eastern Association for the Surgery of Trauma (EAST) released guidelines recommending upper cervical CT (occiput-C3) for evaluation of these patients. Despite this there was very limited data regarding the benefits of this new approach, especially in light of its potential costs, including increased radiation and expense.

OBJECTIVES
To prospectively compare the 1998 EAST guidelines recommending cervical CT to traditional plain films for the evaluation of cervical spine injury in patients with blunt trauma and AMS.

METHODS
Prospective, unblinded, consecutive series at an urban university hospital during a 12-month period between 1998 and 1999.

Participants
1,356 blunt trauma patients, >14 years old, with AMS and requiring CT scan of ≥ two body systems. Select exclusion criteria: Death or clinically cleared before plain films were obtained.

Interventions
All included patients first underwent upper cervical CT and then underwent five-view cervical spine plain film series (lateral, anteroposterior, odontoid, and bilateral, oblique views) after hemodynamic stabilization.

Outcomes
Primary outcome was presence of cervical spine injury on final dictated radiographic diagnosis by two unblinded attending radiologists.

KEY RESULTS
- 5.2% of patients (70) had a total of 95 cervical spine injuries with several sustaining multiple injuries.
- Among those with injuries CT identified 96% (67/70), plain film identified 54% (38/70).
- Seventeen percent (12/70) had neurologic deficits attributable to injuries of the upper cervical spine.
- Among the three patients with a false-negative CT, one had a significant neurologic deficit; among the 32 patients with false-negative plain films, four had significant neurologic deficits.

STUDY CONCLUSIONS
CT scan of cervical spine was superior to five-view plain films in the early identification of upper cervical spine injury in the evaluation of blunt trauma patients with AMS.

COMMENTARY
There has been a transition toward increased use of CT for blunt trauma patients during the past decade as CT scanners have become ubiquitous; however, it was not clear if the use of CT improved the diagnosis of injuries for body systems otherwise well imaged on plain radiography, such as the cervical spine. Although focusing on the upper cervical spine only, this early study was one of the first trials to evaluate this practice and to assess the accuracy of CT vs. plain films in patients with AMS, a population unable to participate in a reliable clinical history and examination necessary for use of clinical decision rules such as NEXUS or the Canadian C-spine Rules. While some providers continue to advocate cervical plain films, this study makes it clear that the standard of care should be cervical CT for this higher-risk trauma population and trauma guidelines continue to recommend this approach.

Question
Is CT imaging of the cervical spine in trauma patients more accurate than plain film radiography for detecting injuries?

Answer
Yes, CT imaging detects significantly more cervical spine injuries than plain films in blunt trauma patients with altered mental status.

CHAPTER 93
THE NEXUS CRITERIA AND THE CANADIAN C-SPINE RULES

Validity of a Set of Clinical Criteria to Rule Out Injury to the Cervical Spine in Patients with Blunt Trauma. National Emergency X-Radiography Utilization Study Group
Hoffman JR, Mower WR, Wolfson AB, Todd KH, Zucker MI. *N Engl J Med.* 2000; 343(2):94–99

The Canadian C-Spine Rule for Radiography in Alert and Stable Trauma Patients
Stiell IG, Wells GA, Vandemheen KL, et al. *JAMA.* 2001;286(15):1841–1848

BACKGROUND

More than 14 million patients undergo radiographic imaging of the c-spine each year in the United States. In less than 2% of all cases a clinically significant spine or cord injury is identified. Prior to the development of validated clinical decision rules there was an excessive use of c-spine imaging in patients with blunt trauma due in part to the high morbidity and medicolegal risk associated with missed c-spine fractures. The NEXUS criteria were validated first, and while highly sensitive for injury, some criticized that they were not specific enough and did not include mechanism of injury in the evaluation. These were followed closely by the development of the Canadian C-Spine Rules.

OBJECTIVES

Both studies sought to create a clinical guideline that could identify patients with minor trauma in whom c-spine computed tomography (CT) could safely be avoided. The Canadian study also attempted to identify those at high risk of c-spine injury.

	NEXUS Criteria	Canadian C-Spine Rule
Methods	Prospective observational study at 21 centers across the United States. Dates not given.	A prospective cohort study occurring in 10 Canadian EDs from 1996–1999.
Participants	34,069 patients who sustained blunt trauma and had c-spine radiographs in the ED. Ages ranged from <1–101 yr with 2.5% <8 yr old.	8,924 alert and stable adult trauma patients who had sustained acute, blunt trauma to the head or neck with potential for cervical spine injury. Convenience sample.
Intervention	Standard series of three views of the c-spine were obtained unless CT or MRI was performed. The decision rule was compared with all imaging. Follow-up review of neurosurgical records for 3 mo to identify missed clinically significant injuries.	Clinical criteria evaluated at the time of attending physician assessment for suspected cervical spine injury. Patients receiving radiography had either plain films, CT, or flexion/extension films, as determined by the treating physician. Patients who did not receive radiography were followed with a structured phone interview to determine the possibility of missed cervical spine injuries.

(continued)

Chapter 93 ■ The NEXUS Criteria and the Canadian C-Spine Rules

	NEXUS Criteria	Canadian C-Spine Rule
Outcomes	Primary outcome was diagnosis and type of c-spine injury according to the final interpretation of all imaging studies without knowledge of clinical results.	A number of univariate analysis techniques were used to identify clinical criteria that were predictive of significant cervical spine injury.
KEY RESULTS	• 818 (2.4%) had radiographically documented c-spine injury. • 8/818 were false negatives by the NEXUS criteria, two of which were clinically significant as defined a priori. • Decision tool has sensitivity of 99% and NPV of 99.8% for clinically significant injury. • The decision tool would have decreased radiography by 12.6%.	• 151 (1.7%) had clinically important c-spine injuries. • The derived decision rule was 100% sensitive and 42.63% specific for identifying clinically significant cervical spine injuries. • The derived decision rule would have decreased the radiography rate by 15.8%.
STUDY CONCLU-SIONS	This study confirms the validity of a decision instrument based on five clinical criteria for identifying, with a high degree of confidence, patients with blunt trauma who have an extremely low probability of having sustained injury to the cervical spine.	The Canadian C-Spine Rule was found to be 100% sensitive for identifying clinically significant cervical spine injuries and has the potential to decrease the rate of unnecessary cervical spine imaging in alert, stable blunt trauma patients.

COMMENTARY

These studies were the first, and remain the most widely used, clinical decision rules to evaluate for cervical spine injury in the trauma patient. These two sets of independently developed clinical decision rules allow for selective use of imaging in patients with suspected cervical fractures. In 2003, a head-to-head study was performed to compare these two rules. The Canadian C-Spine Rule is more specific than the NEXUS and leads to less unnecessary imaging. However, a limitation of the Canadian C-Spine Rule is physicians' unwillingness to rotate the head, thus precluding its effectiveness at the patient's bedside. When compared to Canadian C-Spine Rule, NEXUS is easier to use and ranks higher with regard to physician comfort and appropriate use; however, fewer imaging studies are avoided. This has led some experts to recommend NEXUS criteria to be applied as a first step in the ED. Hence even though both clinical decision rules are endorsed in many international guidelines individually, a stepwise application has been recommended as a way to potentially optimize diagnostic accuracy in blunt trauma patients.

Question

Can cervical spine injury safely be excluded in trauma patients without imaging?

Answer

Yes, both the NEXUS criteria and the Canadian Cervical Spine Rule can safely rule out the need for imaging in stable patients with blunt trauma in whom there is a low clinical suspicion for a cervical spine injury.

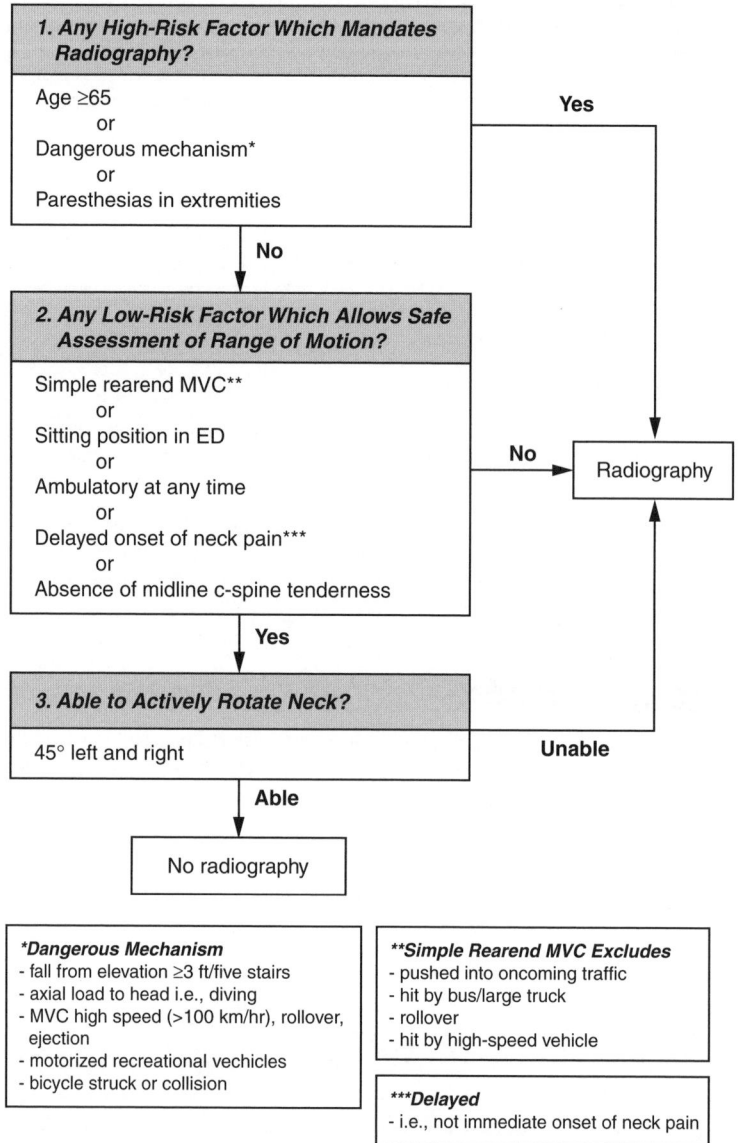

Figure 93.1 Canadian C-Spine Rule. (From Stiell IG, Clement CM, McKnight RD, et al. The Canadian C-Spine rule vs. the NEXUS low-risk criteria in patients with trauma. *New Engl J Med*. 2003;349:2510–2518.)

Table 93.1 The NEXUS Low-risk Criteria[a]

Cervical spine radiography is indicated for patients with trauma unless they meet all of the following criteria:
  No posterior midline cervical spine tenderness,[b]
  No evidence of intoxication,[c]
  A normal level of alertness,[d]
  No focal neurologic deficit,[e] and
  No painful distracting injuries.[f]

From Stiell IG, Clement CM, McKnight RD, et al. The Canadian C-Spine rule vs. the NEXUS low-risk criteria in patients with trauma. *New Engl J Med*. 2003;349:2510–2518.

[a]Criteria are from Hoffman JR, Mower WR, Wolfson AB, Todd KH, Zucker MI. Validity of a set of clinical criteria to rule out injury to the cervical spine in patients with blunt trauma. National Emergency X-Radiography Utilization Study Group. *N Engl J Med* 2000;343:94–99 [Erratum, *N Engl J Med* 2001;344:464.]

[b]Midline posterior bony cervical spine tenderness is present if the patient reports pain on palpation of the posterior midline neck from the nuchal ridge to the prominence of the first thoracic vertebra, or if the patient evinces pain with direct palpation of any cervical spinous process.

[c]Patients should be considered intoxicated if they have either of the following: A recent history provided by the patient or an observer of intoxication or intoxicating ingestion, or evidence of intoxication on physical examination such as an odor of alcohol, slurred speech, ataxia, dysmetria, or other cerebellar findings, or any behavior consistent with intoxication. Patients may also be considered to be intoxicated if tests of bodily secretions are positive for alcohol or drugs that affect the level of alertness.

[d]An altered level of alertness can include any of the following: A Glasgow Coma Scale score of 14 or less; disorientation to person, place, time, or events; an inability to remember three objects at 5 minutes; a delayed or inappropriate response to external stimuli; or other findings.

[e]A focal neurologic deficit is any focal neurologic finding on motor or sensory examination.

[f]No precise definition of a painful distracting injury is possible. This category includes any condition thought by the clinician to be producing pain sufficient to distract the patient from a second (neck) injury. Such injuries may include, but are not limited to, any long-bone fracture; a visceral injury requiring surgical consultation; a large laceration, degloving injury, or crush injury; large burns; or any other injury causing acute functional impairment. Physicians may also classify any injury as distracting if it is thought to have the potential to impair the patient's ability to appreciate other injuries.

CHAPTER 94
NEW ORLEANS CRITERIA AND THE CANADIAN HEAD CT RULES

Indications for Computed Tomography in Patients with Minor Head Injury
Haydel MJ, Preston CA, Mills TJ, Luber S, Blaudeau E, DeBlieux PM. et al. *N Engl J Med.* 2000;343(2):100–105

The Canadian CT Head Rule for Patients with Minor Head Injury
Stiell IG, Wells GA, Vandemheen K, et al. *Lancet.* 2001;357:1391–1396

BACKGROUND
Prior to 2000 there was no validated set of clinical criteria to guide the use of head computed tomography (CT) in patients with minor head injury. In 2000, the first decision tool coined the New Orleans Criteria (NOC) was derived and validated, followed closely in 2001 by the Canadian CT Head Rule (CCHR). There was significant debate regarding which rule was superior due to distinct measures and different primary outcome measures. Criticism of the NOC focused on poor ability to decrease CT scans while the CCHR was criticized for lower sensitivity.

OBJECTIVES
Both studies sought to create a clinical guideline that could identify patients with minor head injury in whom CT head could safely be avoided.

	New Orleans Criteria	Canadian CT Head Rule
Methods	Prospective study in a Level 1 trauma center from 1997 to 1999. Included derivation phase and validation phase.	Prospective cohort study at 10 Canadian hospitals from 1996 to 1999.
Participants	1,429 patients, 3–97 year old, who presented within 24 hour of blunt head trauma with a normal neurologic examination and a Glasgow Coma Scale (GCS) score of 15.	3,121 patients, 16–99 year old, who presented within 24 hour of blunt head injury with loss of consciousness (LOC), amnesia or disorientation, and initial GCS ≥13.
Intervention	All participants had head CT. In phase 1, eight *a priori* clinical factors were evaluated prior to head CT. In phase 2 the guideline derived in phase 1 was compared to CT findings with radiologists blinded.	Standard head CT was done at the discretion for treating physician. EM physicians assessed for 22 standardized clinical variables. 14-day follow-up by telephone and recall if necessary.
Outcomes	Primary outcome – presence of an acute traumatic intracranial lesion (subdural, epidural, or parenchymal hematoma; subarachnoid hemorrhage; cerebral contusion; or depressed skull fracture) on CT scan.	Primary outcome – need for neurological intervention (death or neurosurgical procedure). Secondary outcome – clinically important brain injury requiring hospital admission or neurologic follow-up.

(continued)

	New Orleans Criteria	Canadian CT Head Rule
Key Results	• Final clinical criteria included the following seven variables: Age >60, vomiting, drug or alcohol intoxication, short-term memory loss, seizure after the injury, and evidence of trauma above the clavicles. • The presence of any one of the seven factors yielded a decision rule with a sensitivity of 100%, a negative predictive value (NPV) of 100%, and a specificity of 25% for a positive scan. • None of the patients who required neurosurgical intervention would have been missed with the NOC. • The implementation of the decision rule would have led to a 22% reduction in the use of CT.	• The CCHR is composed of five high-risk factors: GCS <15 at 2 hrs after injury, suspected open or depressed skull fracture, any sign of basal skull fracture, vomiting ≥ two episodes, age ≥65, and two medium-risk factors: Amnesia >30 min and dangerous mechanism. • The presence of any one of the five high-risk factors were 100% sensitive and 68.7% specific for predicting need for neurologic intervention, and would require 32% of patients to undergo CT. • The presence of any one of the seven factors were 98.4% sensitive and 49.6% specific for predicting clinically important brain injury, and would require 54% of patients to undergo CT. • The rule missed 4 (0.1%) patients with clinically important brain injury but did not miss any patients who required neurosurgical intervention.
Study Conclusions	For the evaluation of patients with minor head injury, the use of CT can be safely limited to those who have at least one of the seven New Orleans Criteria.	The Canadian CT Head rule is a highly sensitive decision rule that can optimize the use of CT in patients with minor head injury.

COMMENTARY

These studies resulted in the first validated clinical decision rules to help guide clinicians assessment of the need for CT imaging in minor head injury patients. The introduction of the NOC and CCHR was followed by significant debate between clinicians seeking to use both. In 2005 there was a direct comparison study. This study demonstrated that both decision tools are highly sensitive for ruling out the most significant traumatic injuries, and the conventional wisdom that the CCHR can more effectively reduce CT imaging without missing clinical significant injuries is true. However, clinicians should be cautious that clinically significant injuries (i.e., requiring neurosurgical intervention) may not be the same as injuries requiring clinical detection, which the NOC are more likely to identify. Based on this study the American College of Emergency Physicians (ACEP) recommends using each for distinct patient populations. Since the NOC specifically enrolled patients with LOC, the policy recommends using this decision rule specifically for those patients. Equally, the CCHR enrolled patients with and without LOC and, therefore, ACEP recommends its use in patients without LOC.

Question

Can intracranial injuries be safely excluded in trauma patients without imaging?

Answer

Yes, both the New Orleans Criteria and the Canadian CT Head Rule can safely exclude clinically significant injuries. The New Orleans Criteria are more sensitive for detecting injuries, while the Canadian CT Head Rule can reduce the use of CT imaging.

High Risk (for Neurologic Intervention)
1. GCS score <15 at 2 hrs after injury
2. Suspected open or depressed skull fracture
3. Any sign of basal skull fracture*
4. Vomiting ≥ two episodes
5. Age ≥65

Medium Risk (for Brain Injury on CT)
6. Amnesia before impact ≥30 min
7. Dangerous mechanism** (*pedestrian, occupant ejected, fall from elevation*)

*Signs of Basal Skull Fracture
- hemotympanum, 'racoon' eyes, CSF otorrhea/rhinorrhea, Battle sign

**Dangerous Mechanism
- pedestrian struck by vehicle
- occupant ejected from motor vehicle
- fall from elevation ≥3 ft or five stairs

Rule Not Applicable If:
- Nontrauma cases
- GCS <13
- Age <16
- Coumadin or bleeding disorder
- Obvious open skull fracture

Figure 94.1 Canadian CT Head Rule. (From Stiell IG, Wells GA, Vandemheen K, et al. The Canadian CT Head Rule for patients with minor head injury. *Lancet.* 2001;357:1391–1396.)

Table 94.1 New Orleans Criteria for Determining if CT is Indicated After Minor Head Injury[a]

CT is needed if the patient meets one or more of the following criteria:
Headache
Vomiting
Age older than 60
Drug or alcohol intoxication
Persistent anterograde amnesia (deficits in short-term memory)
Visible trauma above the clavicle
Seizure

[a]Applicable for adults with a normal Glasgow Coma Scale score of 15 and blunt head trauma that occurred within the previous 24 hours that caused loss of consciousness, definite amnesia, or witnessed disorientation.

CHAPTER 95 ED THORACOTOMIES

Critical Analysis of Two Decades of Experience with Postinjury Emergency Department Thoracotomy in a Regional Trauma Center
Branney SW, Moore EE, Feldhaus KM, Wolfe RE. *J Trauma.* 1998;45(1):87–94

BACKGROUND
Emergency department thoracotomy (EDT) is a life-saving procedure when performed for the appropriate indications. Despite this, indiscriminate use results in increased cost and exposes health care providers to significant occupational risk. Prior to this study, there was no clear pathway to guide the use of EDT and many patients in extremis were treated with futile thoracotomy.

OBJECTIVES
Evaluate outcomes in patients receiving EDT based on the presence or absence of vital signs (VSs) and the mechanism of injury.

METHODS
Retrospective chart review in a US regional Level 1 trauma center between 1974 and 1997.

Patients
868 patients who underwent EDT and had complete medical records in a 23-year period. Blunt trauma accounted for 45%, Gun shot wound (GSW) 38%, and stab wounds stab wound (SWs) for 17%. Prehospital information was available for all patients after 1980 (n = 590).

Intervention Evaluated
Before 1985, data was collected in a log maintained by one of the authors. After 1985, the ICD-9-CM coding for EDT and computerized ED procedure logs were reviewed in conjunction with the author's log. EDT was defined as those procedures performed in the ED during the initial resuscitation of the acutely injured patient. Presence of VS was defined as the presence of a palpable pulse or measured blood pressure.

Outcome
The primary outcome was survival to hospital discharge. The secondary outcome was a cost-benefit analysis of EDT.

KEY RESULTS
- Overall survival was 5% (n = 41). Neurologically intact survivors represented 4% (n = 34). Of the neurologically intact survivors 88% (n = 30) had penetrating injuries and 22% (n = 4) sustained blunt trauma.

- When field VSs were present 2.5% of patients with blunt trauma survived neurologically intact compared to 16.4% with penetrating trauma.
- No patients who sustained blunt trauma and were without VS in the field survived neurologically intact.
- Despite the absence of VS in the field, 9 patients (3.6%) who sustained penetrating injury survived neurologically intact.
- The benefit-charge ratio for the initial costs of patients who sustained EDT was 5.6:1. The benefit-charge ratio decreased to 1.8:1 once the lifelong costs of caring for patients who sustained neurologic impairment after the injury were accounted.

STUDY CONCLUSION

EDT is efficacious and cost-effective for patients who sustain penetrating injury to the thorax despite the presence or absence of VS. In patients with penetrating trauma with injuries outside the thorax consideration to perform an EDT should be based on the presence of a palpable pulse or blood pressure on arrival to the ED. In blunt trauma, EDT should be considered only if the patient has VS in the field and in the ED.

COMMENTARY

EDT can be a life-saving intervention; however, its use is rare and complicated by the need to select those patients for whom this costly and potentially dangerous procedure is beneficial. This single-center, retrospective chart review may not be generalizable and its results may be hampered by misclassification and incomplete data; however, given the challenge in studying such a rare procedure, the authors assemble an impressively large cohort who underwent EDT and help elucidate a more rational clinical pathway for EDT. A major contribution of the study is that it clearly defines in whom EDT should be performed, as well as those in whom further attempts are futile. As described above, the overall survival of EDT is best for isolated penetrating injuries to the heart, and the worst survivals are seen in blunt trauma arrest. Given the preponderance of blunt trauma in comparison to penetrating trauma, this work resulted in fewer and fewer EDT being performed and the ultimate decision by the Emergency Medicine (EM) Residency Review Committee to remove EDT as a required procedure in EM training.

Question

Is there any evidence-based indication for performing a thoracotomy in the ED?

Answer

Yes, an ED thoracotomy is not considered futile in pulseless patients with penetrating injuries to the chest. An ED thoracotomy should only be considered in those patients with blunt trauma or penetrating injuries outside of the thorax who lose vital signs or cardiac activity after being brought to the ED.

CHAPTER 96: PEDIATRIC HEAD TRAUMA

Identification of Children at Very Low Risk of Clinically Important Brain Injuries After Head Trauma: A Prospective Cohort Study
Kuppermann N, Holmes JF, Dayan PS, et al. *Lancet.* 2009;374(9696):1160–1170

BACKGROUND
Many children present after head injury and may be at risk for clinically important traumatic brain injury (TBI). Head computed tomography (CT) is useful to assess for injury; however, there is significant concern about the long-term malignancy risks associated with ionizing radiation in young children. Despite clinical decision rules such as the New Orleans Criteria and the Canadian Head CT Rules for adults, no rule existed to assist in avoiding unnecessary CT scans in children.

OBJECTIVES
To derive and validate an age-specific clinical decision rule to identify pediatric patients with head injury at very low risk for clinically important TBI (ciTBI) thereby avoiding the need for a head CT.

METHODS
Multicenter, prospective, cohort derivation and validation study at 25 EDs within PECARN, a pediatric research network in the United States, between 2004 and 2006.

Patients
42,412 pediatric patients, <18 years old, presenting <24 hours from injury with Glasgow Coma Scale (GCS) of 1–15. The derivation cohort included 8,592 patients <2 years old and 25,283 ≥2 years old and the validation cohort included 2,216 patients <2 years old and 6,411 ≥2 years old.

Interventions
Age-specific clinical decision rules were developed using logistic regression from the derivation cohort and were then validated in a second smaller validation cohort. Clinical variables in the decision rules include mental status and impression of normal behavior by parents, loss of consciousness, severity of injury mechanism, and presence of scalp hematoma, skull fracture, headache, and signs of basilar skull fracture or vomiting. Follow-up calls were conducted at 7 and 90 days to identify all clinically important injuries.

Outcomes
Presence of ciTBI, defined as TBI on CT associated with death from TBI, need for neurosurgery, intubation >24 hours, or hospital admission ≥ two nights.

KEY RESULTS
- Derivation cohort – CT scans were obtained in 14,969 patients (35.3%); ciTBIs occurred in 376 (0.9%) and 60 (0.1%) underwent neurosurgery. Among those not imaged, 5 were found to have ciTBI on follow-up.
- Prediction rule <2 years: Negative predictive value (NPV) for ciTBI of 100% (1,176/1,176); sensitivity of 100% (25/25).
- Prediction rule ≥2 years: NPV of 99.95% (3,798/3,800); sensitivity of 96.8% (61/63).

STUDY CONCLUSIONS
Use of the highly accurate clinical decision rules derived and validated in this study will significantly decrease unnecessary CT use and ionizing radiation exposure in children with low risk of ciTBI.

COMMENTARY
This study is a landmark trial which allows providers to apply rigorous and accurate clinical prediction rules to their pediatric patients with minor head trauma and thereby decrease unnecessary head CT scans. This is especially important in the context of increasing emphasis on reducing ionizing radiation exposure in pediatric patients and builds on prior similar clinical decision rules which were developed for adults. This study provides the first prediction rule for <2 years old preverbal patients, a population at the highest risk from radiation but unable to effectively communicate, therefore, at the highest risk of being scanned unnecessarily. The application of this clinical decision rule is somewhat limited by a reliance on some subjective measures such as a parent's impressions of whether the patient is acting normally. In addition to the important prediction rules this study also helped establish the PECARN network as an important research collaborative which has subsequently investigated several similar important clinical questions.

Question
Can intracranial injuries be safely excluded without CT imaging in pediatric patients with minor head trauma?

Answer
Yes, distinct clinical decision rules can be used with high sensitivity for low-risk children <2 and ≥2 years of age to safely exclude clinically important traumatic brain injuries.

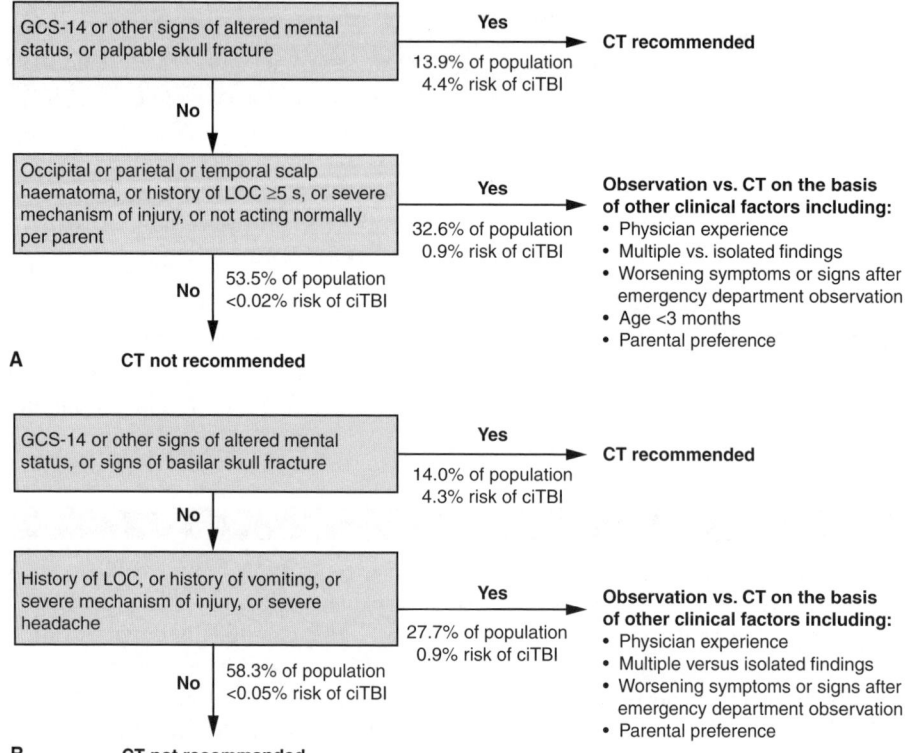

Figure 96.1 Suggested CT algorithm for children less than 2 years old with GCS 14-15 after head trauma.

SECTION 16
ULTRASOUND

Christina Wilson ■ Daphne Morrison Ponce

97. Point of Care Echo in Penetrating Cardiac Injury
98. The Importance of Ultrasound in CVL Placement
99. Ultrasound in Trauma
100. Ultrasound for Resuscitation Termination

CHAPTER 97: POINT OF CARE ECHO IN PENETRATING CARDIAC INJURY

Emergency Department Echocardiography Improves Outcome in Penetrating Cardiac Injury

Plummer D, Brunette D, Asinger R, Ruiz E. *Ann Emerg Med.* 1992;21(6):709–712

BACKGROUND
Prior to the availability of ultrasonography in the ED, the diagnosis of penetrating cardiac injury was made clinically using physical examination and chest x-ray. This often led to delayed and missed diagnosis and resultant high mortality. To improve survival, which requires definitive operative repair, a more rapid and accurate diagnostic test was needed. In 1984 two-dimensional echocardiography, which allows for rapid assessment for pericardial fluid at the bedside, began to be used in EDs. At the time of this paper its impact was not yet known.

OBJECTIVES
To determine the effect of immediate cardiac ultrasound (echo) on time to diagnosis, survival rate, and neurologic outcome in patients presenting to the ED with penetrating cardiac injury.

METHODS
Retrospective chart review at a large regional trauma center between 1980 and 1990.

Participants
Forty-nine trauma patients with penetrating cardiac injury or great vessel injury proven either at operation or autopsy. Twenty-eight had received immediate bedside echo and twenty one had not. Specific characteristics of these two groups are not reported.

Intervention Evaluated
Immediate two-dimensional echo for the presence of pericardial fluid vs. standard assessment.

Outcomes
Survival rate, presumably to hospital discharge but not clearly defined; time to diagnosis in minutes; and neurologic outcomes measured by Glasgow Outcome Score (GOS) at time of discharge of patients with penetrating cardiac injury.

KEY RESULTS
- Survival was 100% in the echo group and 57.1% in the nonecho group.
- The calculated probability of survival based on Injury Severity Score (ISS), age, sex, mechanism, and location of injury was 34.2% for the echo group and 31.8% for the nonecho group.

- The average time to diagnosis was 15.5 ± 11.4 minutes for the echo group and 42.4 ± 21.7 minutes for the nonecho group.
- The Glasgow Outcome Score was 5 for the echo group and 4.2 for the nonecho group.

STUDY CONCLUSIONS

Patients with penetrating cardiac injury who were evaluated with immediate two-dimensional echo had decreased time to diagnosis, improved survival, and improved neurologic outcome than those who were diagnosed clinically.

COMMENTARY

When ultrasound was initially introduced to the ED, it was a novel tool that lacked much evidence demonstrating its impact on emergency care diagnosis and treatment of time-sensitive diseases. Not only did this study show that echo can improve diagnostic capabilities and survival in patients with a traumatic injury that carries a high mortality, but it also provided evidence that an examination routinely performed by cardiologists and trained ultrasonographers can be employed by emergency physicians. Given this study was nonrandomized and retrospective in design these findings may be the results of selection bias or other advances in care other than introduction of echo. Ultimately, this was one of the first studies investigating the use of ED ultrasonography that led the way for many other indications both in trauma and nontraumatic diseases. Based on this study and others, echo has become a key component of the FAST examination and is the standard of care in the evaluation of trauma patients.

Question

Does point-of-care echocardiography on patients presenting to the ED with penetrating cardiac injury improve outcomes?

Answer

Yes, the use of bedside echocardiography may improve survival and decrease time to diagnosis and definitive surgical intervention.

CHAPTER 98
THE IMPORTANCE OF ULTRASOUND IN CENTRAL VENOUS LINE PLACEMENT

Randomized, controlled clinical trial of point-of-care limited ultrasonography assistance of central venous cannulation: The Third Sonography outcomes Assessment Program (SOAP-3) Trial

Milling TJ Jr, Rose J, Briggs WM, et al. *Crit Care Med.* 2005:33(8):1764–1769

BACKGROUND
Central venous line (CVL) placement is a common ED procedure that had traditionally been performed using landmark guidance; however, many patient factors and anatomical variations make this method prone to complications including bleeding, arterial puncture, vessel laceration, and pneumothorax. Despite the fact that both static and dynamic ultrasounds were thought to be beneficial in CVL placement and that the Agency for Healthcare Research and Quality recommended that all CVL placements be done using real-time (dynamic) ultrasound guidance, there was little evidence to support this in the ED.

OBJECTIVES
To compare the efficiency and safety of static ultrasound, dynamic ultrasound, and landmark technique during internal jugular CVL placement.

METHODS
Prospective randomized study at an urban teaching hospital between September 2003 and February 2004.

Patients
Two hundred and one patients with any indication for CVL placement. Select exclusion criteria: Contraindications to internal jugular CVL or lack of consent.

Intervention Evaluated
Characteristics of CVL placement were recorded including overall and first-attempt success rate, number of attempts, time to cannulation, arterial puncture, and patients requiring rescue with dynamic ultrasound.

Outcomes
Primary outcome was successful cannulation. Secondary outcomes included first-attempt success, number of attempts, time to placement, and complications. All outcomes were recorded and both were adjusted for pretest difficulty assessment.

Chapter 98 ■ The Importance of Ultrasound in Central Venous Line Placement

KEY RESULTS
- Use of dynamic ultrasound (US) had the highest unadjusted success rate (98%) when compared with static (82%) and landmark-guided (64%) techniques, with an OR of success over landmark technique of 53.5 for dynamic technique and 3 for static technique.
- Static and dynamic had substantially lower mean first-time attempts (1.7 and 1.6, respectively) when compared with landmark guided (3.2).
- Mean time to cannulation and number of attempts was superior in the static (126 seconds and 1.6 attempts) and dynamic (109 seconds and 1.7 attempts) groups when compared to the landmark guided (250 seconds and 3.2 attempts).
- There was no significant difference in complications between the three groups. All complications were carotid puncture (eight landmark, two dynamic, and two static).

STUDY CONCLUSIONS
Ultrasound guidance with dynamic or static technique is superior to landmark technique for CVL placement.

COMMENTARY
The use of ultrasound for procedural guidance, particularly CVL placement, had initially been studied in the ICU setting and been shown to decrease complications, yet the degree to which these findings extended to the ED was unknown. This study showed that both static and dynamic ultrasounds were superior to landmark technique for CVL placement with the dynamic approach slightly superior to static technique.

This study showed a high first-attempt success rate, fewer attempts, and shorter time to CVL placement in the ultrasound groups. Although this study was not able to detect a difference in complication rates between the three groups, the other findings helped lay the foundation for the ACEP guideline which recommends that all providers learn and use ultrasound for CVL placement.

Question
Does the use of ultrasound significantly improve internal jugular (IJ) line placement when compared to the traditional landmark technique?

Answer
Yes, dynamic ultrasound placement is safer and increases success when compared to landmark-guided IJ central venous catheterization.

CHAPTER 99 ULTRASOUND IN TRAUMA

Randomized Controlled Clinical Trial of Point-of-care, Limited Ultrasonography for Trauma in the Emergency Department: The First Sonography Outcomes Assessment Program Trial
Melniker LA, Leibner E, McKenney MG, et al. *Ann Emerg Med.* 2006;48(3):227–235

BACKGROUND
Torso trauma accounts for more than five million ED visits annually, and is the leading cause of death in patients younger than 45 years. Identifying those patients requiring intervention is essential as those with the shortest time to definitive care have the best outcome. At the time of this study, point-of-care, limited ultrasonography (PLUS) had been shown to be accurate in identifying patients with traumatic injury; however, it had not been shown to improve clinical outcomes.

OBJECTIVES
To determine how a focused assessment with sonography for patients in trauma (FAST) affects time to definitive operative care, as well as its effect on CT use, length of stay, hospital charges, and complications.

METHODS
Prospective, randomized trial at two US trauma centers between 2002 and 2003.

Patients
Two hundred and sixty-two of 444 eligible patients were enrolled. All patients in whom torso trauma was suspected were eligible for enrollment. Select exclusion criteria: being transferred directly to the operating room or lack of consent.

Intervention Evaluated
Standard four-view FAST examination was performed in patients randomized to the intervention group.

FAST protocol views: (1) Pericardial space to assess for effusion, (2) right upper quadrant to assess for right hemothorax and fluid in Morrison pouch, (3) left upper quadrant to assess for left hemothorax and fluid in splenorenal recess or left subdiaphragm, and (4) pelvis to assess for fluid in pouch of Douglas or cul-de-sac.

Outcomes
The primary outcome was time from ED arrival to transfer for operative care. Secondary outcomes included use of CT, hospital length of stay, complications, and total charges.

KEY RESULTS
- 29% (63) patients required operative care.
- Transfer to the Operating Room was 64% faster (57 vs. 166 minutes) in the FAST group as compared to the control.
- Point-of-care ultrasound reduced the use of CT in both operative and nonoperative patients.
- Admitted point-of-care ultrasound patients had decreased hospital length of stay (6.2 vs. 10.2 days in operative patients; 10.7 vs. 15.1 in nonoperative patients) as compared to the control.
- Point-of-care ultrasound patients had a reduction in charges of 35%.

STUDY CONCLUSIONS
The use of point-of-care limited ultrasonography in patients with suspected torso trauma results in reduction of time to definitive care.

COMMENTARY
This study reaffirms that the use of FAST in trauma patients is not only accurate when performed by emergency providers, but also improves patients' treatment and outcomes. This study was the first of its kind to both have a randomized design and be powered to detect differences between the groups. This study also looked at the subset of patients not requiring immediate operative intervention, further reinforcing the importance of point-of-care ultrasound. As a result of this and subsequent work, FAST has become a standard of trauma care that has replaced the use of diagnostic peritoneal lavage in the current Advanced Trauma Life Support algorithm. Limitations of this study include that treating physicians were not blinded to the randomization and, therefore, a reduction in time to treatment may have resulted from this awareness. Since this time, emergency provider awareness and skill with point-of-care ultrasound has evolved to include thoracic imaging as well as coordinated plans of care at trauma centers for patients with positive ultrasound findings.

Question
Does the use of ED point-of-care ultrasound for patients with blunt torso trauma improve outcomes?

Answer
Yes, point-of-care ultrasound increases the speed of transfer to the OR and decreases the use of CT imaging, hospital length of stay, and total patient charges.

CHAPTER 100: ULTRASOUND FOR RESUSCITATION TERMINATION

Outcome in Cardiac Arrest Patients Found to Have Cardiac Standstill on the Bedside Emergency Department Echocardiogram

Blaivas M, Fox JC, *Acad Emerg Med.* 2001;8:616–621

BACKGROUND
While clear ACLS guidelines exist for the management of cardiac arrest, there has been limited research to guide the termination of resuscitation for cardiac arrest. For patients who arrive to the ED in cardiac arrest, resuscitation can often continue for prolonged periods of time and require significant resources when electrical activity on the monitor is the only sign of life. At the time of this study, limited bedside echocardiography (echo) had already been shown valuable in evaluating select etiologies in cardiac arrest, but not as a prognostic tool to guide resuscitation efforts.

OBJECTIVES
To evaluate the outcomes of patients presenting to the ED in cardiac arrest with echo confirmed cardiac standstill.

METHODS
Prospective, observational study conducted at a single US academic ED between 1999 and 2000.

Participants
Convenience sample of 173 patients presenting with ongoing CPR to an urban, community ED with resident staffing.

Intervention Evaluated
Each enrolled patient had a rapid bedside echocardiogram performed upon transfer from EMS stretcher to ED bed during pulse check. A single subxiphoid, four-chamber view was obtained. All bedside echos were performed by ultrasound trained and credentialed emergency physicians. Summary arrest data including downtime, time without and with CPR, and ACLS measures used were collected from EMS personnel and family when possible. Patients were defined to be in asystole if no myocardial contractions were seen for the duration of a pulse check, and death was confirmed with a 20-second echo after declaration of death.

Outcomes
The primary outcome was survival to hospital admission. Survival from cardiac arrest was defined as return of spontaneous circulation in the ED without any additional electrical shocks or medical interventions.

KEY RESULTS
- One hundred and seventy-three of a possible 800 patients presenting with ongoing CPR were enrolled and bedside echo was performed in 169 patients without evidence of interference in resuscitative efforts.
- Cardiac standstill on initial echo had a 100% PPV for death in the ED regardless of initial rhythm.
- 11.8% of patients (20) survived to hospital admission, none demonstrated cardiac standstill on echo at ED presentation.
- All patients presenting with asystole on rhythm strip or EKG (38%; 65 patients) had cardiac standstill on ultrasound.

STUDY CONCLUSIONS
Patients presenting to the ED with cardiac standstill on bedside echo uniformly did not survive to hospital admission regardless of initial rhythm.

COMMENTARY
There is a large body of literature used to support the ACLS protocols that guide the management of patients with cardiac arrest, yet limited guidance on when to terminate these resuscitations. The traditional clinical examination findings of death are neither easy nor possible to utilize during active CPR, resulting in frequently prolonged and futile resuscitations that require considerable ED resources. This study showed a 100% PPV for death for patients with cardiac standstill on bedside echo regardless of the rhythm identified on the monitor—a finding that can be easily and quickly detected by even novice users of bedside echo and requires no associated clinical history or examination information. These findings should be interpreted with some caution as the study included only a convenience sample of less than 20% of cardiac arrests arriving at the study site, and all echoes were performed by unblinded study authors with advanced ultrasound training. This study demonstrates the broadening use of bedside ultrasound across nontraumatic uses in the ED and the potential for ultrasound to provide definitive prognostic information. Although more communities are developing protocols for field termination of cardiac arrest, many patients with equivocal downtime, family preference or local care patterns continue to be evaluated in the ED and require rapid assessment to distinguish between those with survivable vs. terminal cardiac arrest.

Question
Can bedside ultrasound be used to guide the termination of CPR?

Answer
Yes, in patients with cardiac standstill on bedside echo at ED arrival there is no chance of survival to hospital admission.

INDEX

Note: Page locator followed by f and t indicates figure and table respectively.

A

AAP. *See* American Academy of Pediatrics (AAP)
ABCD score, 132–133, 134t
Abdominal GSW. *See* Gunshot wounds (GSW)
Abdominal pain
  clinically significant diagnostic accuracy, 158
  clinically significant diagnostic error, 158
  morphine administration for, 158–159
ABG. *See* Arterial blood gas (ABG)
Abnormal neurologic status, 208
ABS. *See* Agitated behavior scale (ABS)
ACEP. *See* American College of Emergency Physicians (ACEP)
Acetaminophen, 122
  hepatotoxicity, 206
  and N-acetylcysteine, 204, 206–207
  plasma acetaminophen concentrations, 206
  poisoning, 204–205
  Rumack and Matthew observation, 204–205
  toxicity, 204–205
ACS. *See* Acute coronary syndrome (ACS)
Acute coronary syndrome (ACS), 40
  with elevated troponin, 54
  and percutaneous intervention timing, 54–55
  without ST-segment elevation, 54
Acute myocardial infarction (MI), 18–19, 38–39
  aspirin in, 46–47
  beta-blockers in, 44–45
  fibrinolytic therapy, 44
  heparin, 50, 51
  ISIS-2, 46, 47
  streptokinase, 50, 51
  tissue plasminogen activator (tPA), 50–52
Acute otitis media (AOM)
  antibiotic prescription, 104
  treatment of, 104
  wait-and-see prescription approach, 104–105
Acute respiratory distress syndrome (ARDS), 184–185
Acyclovir, 118–119
AFib. *See* Atrial fibrillation (AFib)
Agitated behavior scale (ABS), 180
Alcohol dehydrogenase, 200
Alcohol Use Disorders Identification Test (AUDIT), 148
Alertness scale, 180
Allergic syndromes
  H_2-blockers, 32
  histamine antagonists in, 32–33
  IV diphenhydramine, 32
  IV ranitidine, 32
Alteplase, 130
Altered mental status (AMS), 222
American Academy of Pediatrics (AAP), 12
American College of Emergency Physicians (ACEP), 229
AMI. *See* Acute myocardial infarction (AMI)
Amiodarone, 66–67
Amoxicillin, 94
AMS. *See* Altered mental status (AMS)
Analgesia, 158, 160, 162, 163
Anaphylaxis, 212
Angioedema, 32
Angioplasty, 52
Ankle injuries, 154
Antithrombotics
  heparin, 52
  hirudin, 52
Antivenom, 212–213
AOM. *See* Acute otitis media (AOM)
Apnea, 24, 25
Appendectomy, 2
Appendicitis, 2–3
ARDS. *See* Acute respiratory distress syndrome (ARDS)
Arterial blood gas (ABG), 82
  vs. pulse oximetry, 196–197
Arterial puncture, 240
Aspartate transaminase (AST), 204
Aspirin, 46–47
AST. *See* Aspartate transaminase (AST)
Asthma. *See also* Bronchospasm
  intravenous magnesium in, 186–187
  ipratropium bromide for, 188
  nebulized salbutamol for, 188
Atrial fibrillation (AFib)
  flecainide, 74
  "Pill-in-the-Pocket" approach, 74–75
  propafenone, 74
  rate control in, 76–77
  rhythm control in, 76–77
  stroke risk in, 78–79
  thromboembolism in, 78–79

247

AUDIT. *See* Alcohol Use Disorders Identification Test (AUDIT)
AV block, 210

B
Backward-upward-rightward pressure (BURP), 26, 27
Bacterial meningitis
  in adult, 94–95
  amoxicillin, 94
  in child, 96–97
  CT scan, 116–117
  dexamethasone in, 94–97
Barthel index, 125
Bell's palsy
  efficacy of acyclovir, 118–119
  efficacy of prednisolone, 118–119
Benign positional vertigo (BPV)
  Epley maneuver for, 138–139
Benzodiazepines, 180
Beta-blockers
  in acute myocardial infarction, 44–45
  fibrinolytic therapy, 44
Beta-lactams, 30
BI. *See* Brief interventions (BI)
Bicarbonate therapy, 84–85
Bimanual laryngoscopy, 26, 27
Bleeding, 240
BNI. *See* Brief negotiation interview (BNI)
Borrelia burgdorferi, 100
BPRS. *See* Brief psychiatric rating scale (BPRS)
BPV. *See* Benign positional vertigo (BPV)
Brief interventions (BI), 148–149
  BNI with booster, 148
  brief negotiation interview, 148
Brief negotiation interview (BNI), 148
Brief psychiatric rating scale (BPRS), 180
Bronchospasm
  intravenous magnesium in, 186–187
  peak expiratory flow rate, 186
BURP. *See* Backward-upward-rightward pressure (BURP)

C
CAD. *See* Coronary artery disease (CAD)
Caffeine, 122
Canadian C-spine rules, 223, 224–225, 226f
  vs. NEXUS criteria, 226f
Canadian CT head rule (CCHR), 228–229
CAP. *See* Community-acquired pneumonia (CAP)
Carbon monoxide poisoning
  cognitive sequelae, 202–203
  HBO on, 202–203
  hyperbaric oxygen for, 202

Cardiac arrest
  epinephrine for, 68–69
  with pulseless electrical activity, 70–71
  therapeutic hypothermia in, 60–61
  vasopressin *vs.* epinephrine, 72–73
Cardiac biomarkers, 42
Cardiac ischemia
  missed diagnoses of, 40–41
  myocardial infarctions (MIs), 40
  unstable angina (UA), 40
Cardiopulmonary resuscitation (CPR), 58–59
  by chest compression, 64–65
  in out-of-hospital cardiac arrest, 62–63
CCHR. *See* Canadian CT head rule (CCHR)
CDC. *See* Center for Disease Control (CDC)
Ceftriaxone, 30
Cefuroxime, 30
Cellular hypoxia, 208
Center for Disease Control (CDC), 12
Central line-associated bloodstream infections (CLABSI), 102
  intervention to, 102–103
Central venous line (CVL)
  characteristics
    complications, 240
    first attempt success, 240
    number of attempts, 240
    time to placement, 240
  complications
    arterial puncture, 240
    bleeding, 240
    pneumothorax, 240
    vessel laceration, 240
  ultrasound in, 240–241
Cephalosporins, in penicillin-allergic patients, 30–31
Cerebrospinal fluid (CSF), 96
Cervical spine injuries
  and altered mental status, 222
  in blunt trauma, 222
  computed tomography in, 222–223
  and neurologic deterioration, 222
  plain films in, 222–223
  radiographic diagnosis, 222–223
Cervical spine plain film series views
  anteroposterior, 222
  bilateral, 222
  lateral, 222
  oblique, 222
  odontoid, 222
Cervical spine radiography, 227
  NEXUS low-risk criteria for, 227t
CGI. *See* Clinical global impressions (CGI)
Chest compressions, 64–65

Chest pain, 38
  AMI without, 38–39
  exercise stress test, 144
  length of stay in hospital, 144
  protocol vs hospitalization in patients, 144–145
  troponins in, 42–43
Chest pain variable, 38
Child–Pugh score, 6
Chromaturia, 209
Chronic obstructive pulmonary disease (COPD)
  antibiotics in, 194–195
  corticosteroids in, 192
  oral vs. IV prednisolone, 192–193
  peak expiratory flow rate, 194
ciTBI, 234
  negative predictive value for, 235
CLABSI. See Central line-associated bloodstream infections (CLABSI)
Clinical global impressions (CGI), 180
Community-acquired pneumonia (CAP), 92
Complete portal vein thrombosis, 6
Computed tomographic venous-phase imaging (CTV), 176
Computed tomography (CT), 2
  in cervical spine injuries, 222–223
  for minor head injury, 228–229
  for pulmonary embolism (PE), 176–177
  for traumatic brain injury, 234
Continuous positive airway pressure ventilation (CPAP), 18–19
COPD. See Chronic obstructive pulmonary disease (COPD)
Coronary angioplasty, 52
Coronary artery disease (CAD), 146
Corticosteroids, 190
  in chronic obstructive pulmonary disease, 192
CPAP. See Continuous positive airway pressure ventilation (CPAP)
CPR. See Cardiopulmonary resuscitation (CPR)
Cricoid pressure, 26, 27
Crotalinae polyvalent immune Fab (Fab AV), 212–213
Croup
  corticosteroids for, 190
  oral dexamethasone, 190–191
CSF. See Cerebrospinal fluid (CSF)
CT. See Computed tomography (CT)
CT scan
  for acute appendicitis, 2–3
  for bacterial meningitis, 116–117
  cost, 3
  of head, 116–117
  ureterolithiasis, 10
CTV. See Computed tomographic venous-phase imaging (CTV)

CURB-63 scores, 93
CVL. See Central venous line (CVL)
Cyanide poisoning, 208–209
Cyanide toxicity
  hydroxocobalamin for, 208–209
  morbidity of, 208
  mortality of, 208

D
D-dimer tests
  in deep venous thrombosis
    negative likelihood ratio, 172
    positive likelihood ratio, 172
    sensitivity, 172
    specificity, 172
  in pulmonary embolism
    negative likelihood ratio, 172
    positive likelihood ratio, 172
    sensitivity, 172
    specificity, 172
Deep vein thrombosis (DVT), 166
  D-dimer tests in, 172–173
Dexamethasone, 96–97, 190
Diabetic ketoacidosis (DKA)
  arterial vs. venous blood gas, 82–83
  bicarbonate therapy in, 84–85
Digitalis toxicity
  AV block, 210
  with digoxin-specific fab antibody fragments, 210–211
  ventricular tachycardia, 210
Digoxin toxicity, 210
Dizziness, 138
DKA. See Diabetic ketoacidosis (DKA)
Doxycycline, 100–101
DVT. See Deep vein thrombosis (DVT)
Dysrhythmia, 22, 23

E
Early goal-directed therapy (EGDT), 88
EAST. See Eastern Association for Surgery of Trauma (EAST)
Eastern Association for Surgery of Trauma (EAST), 222
EDT. See Emergency department thoracotomy (EDT)
ED training, rapid sequence intubation in, 22–23
EGDT. See Early goal-directed therapy (EGDT)
ELISA, 173
Emergency department thoracotomy (EDT)
  ICD-9-CM coding for, 232
  mechanism of injury for, 232
  vital signs for, 232–233
Endotracheal intubation, 26

End-tidal carbon dioxide (ETCO$_2$)
   during PSA, 20
   in sedation, 20–21
Enoxaparin, 50, 51
Enoxaparin in non-Q-wave coronary events (ESSENCE), 36
Envenomation syndrome, 212–213
Epinephrine, 68–69
   vs. vasopressin, 72–73
Epley maneuver
   for benign positional vertigo, 138–139
Erythema, 32
Ethanol
   for ethylene glycol poisoning, 200
   side effects
      hepatotoxicity, 200
      hypoglycemia, 200
      intoxication, 200
Ethylene glycol poisoning, 200–201
   ethanol for, 200–201
   fomepizole for, 200–201
   metabolites, 200
   plasma glycolate concentrations, 200–201
   renal injury, 200
   side effects (*See* Ethanol)
   treatment, 200
   urinary oxalate excretion, 200–201
ETT. *See* Exercise treadmill testing (ETT)
Exercise stress test, 144
   EKG monitoring, 144
Exercise treadmill testing (ETT), 146

F

Fab AV. *See* Crotalinae polyvalent immune Fab (Fab AV)
Fab fragments, 210–211
FAST. *See* Focused assessment with sonography for patients in trauma (FAST)
Febrile infants
   Boston criteria, 108–110
   management, 108
   Philadelphia criteria, 108–110
   Rochester criteria, 108–110
   with RSV, 112–113
   serious bacterial infection, 108, 112–113
Flecainide, 74
Focused assessment with sonography for patients in trauma (FAST), 242
   protocol views, 242
   in trauma patients, 243
Fomepizole, 200–201

G

GAS. *See* Group A betahemolytic streptococcus (GAS)

GAS pharyngitis, 106–107
Gastric pH, 5
Gastroenteritis
   oral ondansetron in, 12–13
   oral rehydration therapy in, 14–15
Gastrointestinal bleeding, 4–5
GI bleeding, 8
   nasogastric (NG) aspiration, 8
   NG lavage in, 8
   test characteristics estimation of NG aspiration
      likelihood ratio (LR), 8
      negative predictive value (NPV), 8
      positive predictive value (PPV), 8
      sensitivity, 8
      specificity, 8
Glasgow outcome scale, 94
Glasgow outcome score (GOS), 238
Global use of strategies to open occluded coronary arteries (GUSTO IIB), 52
GOS. *See* Glasgow outcome score (GOS)
Group A betahemolytic streptococcus (GAS), 106–107
GSW. *See* Gunshot wounds (GSW)
Gunshot wounds (GSW)
   laparotomy in, 216–217
   nonoperative management for, 216–217
GUSTO IIB. *See* Global use of strategies to open occluded coronary arteries (GUSTO IIB)

H

Haemophilus influenzae type b, 97
Haloperidol, 180–181
HB. *See* Hyperbaric oxygen (HB)
H$_2$-blockers, 32
Hematemesis
   diagnostic nasogastric aspiration in, 8–9
   NG lavage in, 8
Hemoglobin desaturation, 24–25
Heparin, 48, 51, 52
   for AMI, 50, 51
   for NSTEMI, 49
   for STEMI, 49
Hepatocellular carcinoma, 6
Hepatotoxicity, 200, 206–207
Hirudin, 52
Histamine antagonists, acute allergic syndromes in, 32–33
Horse serum antivenom, 212
   adverse effects
      anaphylaxis, 212
      hypotension, 212
      serum sickness, 212
      urticaria, 212

House–Brackmann grading system, 118
H_2-receptor antagonists, 32
H_2-receptor blockers, 5
Hydrocodone, 122
Hydromorphone, 122–123
Hydroxocobalamin, 208–209
 amelioration of neurologic signs, 208
 hemodynamic characteristics, 208
 neuropsychiatric sequelae, 208
 treatment, 208–209
Hyperbaric oxygen (HB), 202
Hypertension, 209
Hypoglycemia, 200
Hypotension, 22, 23, 212
Hypoxemia, 20, 22, 23

I
IA tPA. *See* Intraarterial prourokinase (IA tPA)
Ibuprofen, 122, 160–161
ICD-9-CM coding, 232
ICH. *See* Intracranial hemorrhage (ICH)
Idiopathic unilateral facial nerve paralysis. *See* Bell's palsy
IM CTX. *See* Intramuscular ceftriaxone (IM CTX)
Injury severity score (ISS), 238
Intoxication, 200
Intraarterial prourokinase (IA tPA), 126–127
Intracranial hemorrhage (ICH), 130–131
Intramuscular ceftriaxone (IM CTX), 108
Intravenous magnesium, 186–187
Ipratropium bromide, 188
Ischemic stroke
 ECASS II trials, 130
 intra-arterial prourokinase for, 126–127
 NIH stroke scale, 124
 tissue plasminogen activator for, 124–125, 128–129, 130–131
ISIS-2, 47
ISS. *See* Injury severity score (ISS)
IV diphenhydramine, 32
IV ranitidine, 32
Ixodes scapularis, 100

J
JCAHO. *See* Joint Commission on Accreditation of Healthcare Organizations (JCAHO)
Joint Commission on Accreditation of Healthcare Organizations (JCAHO), 162

K
Ketorolac, 122, 160–161
Knee pain, 152–153
 radiography of, 152

L
Lactate, 96
Laparotomy, 216–217
 in gunshot wounds, 216–217
Laryngoscopy
 backward-upward-rightward pressure (BURP), 26
 cricoid pressure, 26
 laryngeal view in, 26–27
Length of stay (LOS), 144
Leptospirosis, 100
Level I trauma centers
 costs, 220
 mortality evaluation in, 220–221
 risks of transfer, 220
 vs. nontrauma center, 220–221
Lidocaine, 66
Likelihood ratio (LR), 8, 9
LMWH. *See* Low-molecular-weight heparin (LMWH)
Lorazepam, 180–181
LOS. *See* Length of stay (LOS)
Low-molecular-weight heparin (LMWH), 50
Low tidal volume ventilation, 184–185
LP. *See* Lumbar puncture (LP)
LR. *See* Likelihood ratio (LR)
Lumbar puncture (LP), 116
Lung injury, 184
Lyme disease
 doxycycline in, 100–101
 Ixodes scapularis, 100
 placebo-control trial, 100–101

M
MBPRS. *See* Modified brief psychiatric rating scale (MBPRS)
MedisGroup database, 92
Meperidine, 122
Methemoglobinemia, 208
Metoclopramide, 120–121
MI. *See* Myocardial infarctions (MI)
Midazolam, 23
Migraine
 acetaminophen, 122
 acetaminophen with butalbital, 122
 caffeine, 122
 hydrocodone, 122
 hydromorphone *vs.* metoclopramide, 122–123
 ibuprofen, 122
 ketorolac, 122
 magnesium, 122
 meperidine, 122
 metoclopramide, 120–121
 ondansetron, 122

Migraine (*continued*)
  prochlorperazine, 120–121, 122
  promethazine, 122
  sumatriptan, 122
  treatment, 122–123
Mild-to-moderate dehydration, 12
Minor head injury
  Canadian CT head rule for, 228
  computed tomography in, 228–229
Modified brief psychiatric rating scale (MBPRS), 180
Morbidity, 8
  and ACS, 54
  of cyanide toxicity, 208
  and ethylene glycol poisoning, 200
Morphine, 158–159
Mortality
  and acute lung injury, 184
  and acute pulmonary edema, 18–19
  and ARDS, 184–185
  of cyanide toxicity, 208
  gunshot wounds, 216–217
  and heart failure, 18–19
  with myocardial infarction, 38–39
  and stroke, 132
  thrombolytic strategies
    accelerated tPA with IV heparin, 50
    streptokinase with IV heparin, 50
    streptokinase with subcutaneous heparin, 50
    streptokinase with tPA and IV heparin, 50
  trauma-center care effect on, 220–221
  and variceal bleeding, 6–7
Musculoskeletal pain
  intramuscular ketorolac *vs.* oral ibuprofen in, 160–161
  NSAID, 160
Myocardial infarctions (MI), 40
  aspirin, 48
  heparin, 48
Myocardial infarction without chest pain
  NRMI-2, 38

N
NAC. *See* N-acetylcysteine (NAC)
N-acetylcysteine (NAC), 204, 206–207
Nasogastric aspiration tube, 8
  in hematemesis, 8–9
Nasogastric (NG) aspiration
  likelihood ratio (LR), 8
  negative predictive value (NPV), 8
  positive predictive value (PPV), 8
  sensitivity, 8
  specificity, 8
National Institute of Neurological Disorders and Stroke (NINDS), 128

National Study on the Costs and Outcomes of Trauma (NSCOT), 220
Nebulized beta-agonists, 188
Nebulized salbutamol, 188
Negative predictive value (NPV), 8, 235
Neurologic deterioration, 222
New Orleans criteria (NOC), 228–229, 230t
NEXUS criteria, 224–225
  for cervical spine radiography, 227t
  vs. Canadian C-spine rules, 226f
NG lavage, 8, 9
NIHSS. *See* NIH Stroke Scale (NIHSS)
NIH Stroke Scale (NIHSS), 124
NINDS. *See* National Institute of Neurological Disorders and Stroke (NINDS)
NOC. *See* New Orleans criteria (NOC)
Non-invasive positive pressure ventilation (NPPV), 18–19
Non-invasive ventilation, pulmonary edema in, 18–19
Non–Q-wave myocardial infarction, 50
Nonsteroidal anti-inflammatory (NSAID), 160
Non-ST–segment elevation myocardial infarction (NSTEMI), 36
  heparin for, 49
NPPV. *See* Non-invasive positive pressure ventilation (NPPV)
NPV. *See* Negative predictive value (NPV)
NRMI-2, 38
NSAID. *See* Nonsteroidal anti-inflammatory (NSAID)
NSCOT. *See* National Study on the Costs and Outcomes of Trauma (NSCOT)
NSTEMI. *See* Non-ST–segment elevation myocardial infarction (NSTEMI)

O
OHCA. *See* Out-of-hospital cardiac arrest (OHCA)
Omeprazole, 4
Ondansetron, 12, 122
Oral ondansetron
  in gastroenteritis, 12–13
  vomiting, 12–13
Oral rehydration therapy (ORT)
  failure rate of, 14
  in gastroenteritis, 14
  in mild-to-moderate dehydration, 14
Oral *vs.* intravenous rehydration, 14–15
ORT. *See* Oral rehydration therapy (ORT)
Ottawa foot and ankle rules, 154–155
Ottawa knee rules, 153–154
Out-of-hospital cardiac arrest (OHCA), 58
  CPR quality in, 62–63
Oxygen saturation, 20

P

PAF. *See* Platelet-activating factor (PAF)
Pain and emergency medicine initiative (PEMI) study, 162–163
PCI. *See* Percutaneous intervention (PCI)
PEA. *See* Pulseless electrical activity (PEA)
Peak expiratory flow rate (PEFR), 186–187
 and COPD, 194
Pediatric head trauma, 234–235
Pediatric meningitis
 dexamethasone in, 96
PEFR. *See* Peak expiratory flow rate (PEFR)
Penetrating cardiac injury, 238–239
 cardiac ultrasound (echo) on, 238–239
Penetrating torso injuries (for hypotensive patients)
 aggressive isotonic fluid administration, 218–219
 immediate *vs.* delayed fluid resuscitation for, 218–219
 postoperative complications
  acute renal failure, 218
  ARDS, 218
  coagulopathy, 218
  pneumonia, 218
  sepsis syndrome, 218
  wound infection, 218
Penicillin-allergic patients
 ceftriaxone, 30
 cephalosporins in, 30–31
 IgE-mediated hypersensitivity to, 30
Penicillins, 30
Peptic ulcer disease (PUD), 4–5
 endoscopy for, 4
 omeprazole therapy, 4
 and placebo, 4
 and PPI therapy, 4
PERC. *See* Pulmonary embolism rule-out criteria (PERC)
Percutaneous intervention (PCI)
 in ACS, 54–55
Pharyngitis, 106
PIOPED. *See* Prospective investigation of pulmonary embolism diagnosis (PIOPED)
PIOPED II study, 176
Placebo, 4, 6, 12
Placebo maneuver, 138
Plasma acetaminophen concentrations, 206
Platelet-activating factor (PAF), 96
Platelet function, 4
Pneumothorax, 240
Point-of-care ultrasound, 242–243
PORT score, 92–93
Positive predictive value (PPV), 8
PPI. *See* Proton pump inhibitor (PPI)
PPV. *See* Positive predictive value (PPV)
Prednisolone, 118–119
 in COPD, 192–193
Procedural sedation and analgesia (PSA)
 $ETCO_2$ monitoring, 20
Prochlorperazine, 120–121
Promethazine, 122
Propafenone, 74
Prospective investigation of pulmonary embolism diagnosis (PIOPED), 174–175
Proton pump inhibitor (PPI)
 in peptic ulcer disease, 4–5
PSA. *See* Procedural sedation and analgesia (PSA)
Psychotic agitation
 ABS scores, 181–182
 haloperidol, 181–182
 lorazepam, 181–182
PUD. *See* Peptic ulcer disease (PUD)
Pulmonary angiography, 174, 176
Pulmonary edema
 AMI, 18–19
 CPAP, 18–19
 non-invasive ventilation in, 18–19
 NPPV, 18–19
Pulmonary embolism (PE)
 clinical features, 166–167
 computed tomographic venous-phase imaging, 176
 computed tomography imaging for, 176–177
 D-dimer tests, 172–173
 deep vein thrombosis, 166
 history, 166
 physical examination, 166
 pulmonary angiography, 176
 ventilation and perfusion lung scans (V/Q scan), 174–175
Pulmonary embolism rule-out criteria (PERC), 168–169
 and DVT, 169
Pulseless electrical activity (PEA), 70–71
Pulse oximetry, 20
 vs. arterial blood gas, 196–197

Q

Q-wave MI, 50

R

Radiolucent stones, 10
Rankin scale, 125
Rapid sequence intubation (RSI), 22–23
 in ED training, 22–23
 succinylcholine, 24

Rapid tranquilization (RT), 180
Renal injury, 200–201
Return of spontaneous circulation (ROSC), 58, 60
 and epinephrine, 68–69
ROSC. *See* Return of spontaneous circulation (ROSC)
RSI. *See* Rapid sequence intubation (RSI)
RT. *See* Rapid tranquilization (RT)
Rumack–Matthew nomogram, 204–205

S
"Safe apnea" period, 25
Sclerotherapy, 6
Sedation, end-tidal carbon dioxide ($ETCO_2$), 20–21
Seizure recurrence risk in children, 140–141
 crypogenic group, 140
 symptomatic group, 140
Sellick maneuver, 26
Sensitivity, 8
Sepsis
 early goal-directed therapy in, 88–89
 EGDT protocol, 88
Septic shock, 88–89
Serious bacterial infection (SBI), 108
 definition, 112
 in febrile infants with RSV, 112–113
SIRS. *See* Systemic inflammatory response syndrome (SIRS)
Skin erythema, 209
Snakebite
 crotalinae polyvalent immune Fab (Fab AV), 212–213
 horse serum antivenom, 212
 in United States, 212
Sodium bicarbonate, 84
Somatostatin analogs, 6–7
Specificity, 8
Spontaneous ureteral stone passage
 CT imaging for, 10
 radiography, 10
 ureteral stone location, 10
 ureteral stone size, 10
Stab wounds (SW), 232
Steroids
 in adults with bacterial meningitis, 94–95
 in children with bacterial meningitis, 97
Strep throat in adults, 106–107
Streptokinase, 50, 51
Succinylcholine, 23, 24
 hemoglobin desaturation, 24–25
Sumatriptan, 122
SW. *See* Stab wounds (SW)

Syphilis, 100
Systemic inflammatory response syndrome (SIRS), 88

T
TBI. *See* Traumatic brain injury (TBI)
Therapeutic hypothermia, 60–61
Thromboembolism, 78–79
Thrombolysis in myocardial infarction (TIMI), 36
Thrombolytics, 52
Thrombolytic strategies
 accelerated tPA with IV heparin, 50
 streptokinase with IV heparin, 50
 streptokinase with subcutaneous heparin, 50
 streptokinase with tPA and IV heparin, 50
TIA. *See* Transient ischemic attack (TIA)
TIMI. *See* Thrombolysis in myocardial infarction (TIMI)
TIMI risk score
 non-ST–segment elevation myocardial infarction, 36
 predictor variables, 36–37
 unstable angina, 36
Tissue plasminogen activator (tPA), 52
 in AMI, 50–51
 in cardiac arrest with pulseless electrical activity, 70–71
 for ischemic stroke, 124–125, 129–130
TNF-alpha, 96
tPA. *See* Tissue plasminogen activator (tPA)
Transient ischemic attack (TIA)
 ABCD score, 132–133
 stroke risk with, 132
 treatment after, 136–137
Traumatic brain injury (TBI)
 clinical decision rule, 234–235
 CT scan for, 234–235, 236f
Troponin I, 42, 43
Troponins
 biomarkers, 42
 in chest pain, 42–43
Troponin T, 42, 43
Two-dimensional echocardiography, 238

U
UA. *See* Unstable angina (UA)
UFH. *See* Unfractioned heparin (UFH)
Ultrasonography, 238
 in central venous line placement, 240–241
 for resuscitation termination, 244–245
 in trauma, 242–243
Unfractioned heparin (UFH), 50
 enoxaparin, 50–51
Unstable angina (UA), 36, 40, 48

Ureterolithiasis, 10–11
  CT scan, 10
Urticaria, 32, 212

V
Vapreotide, 6, 7
Variceal bleeding
  mortality, 6
  sclerotherapy, 6
  somatostatin in, 6–7
Vasopressin, 72
  vs. epinephrine, 72–73
VBG. *See* Venous blood gas (VBG)
Venous blood gas (VBG), 82

Ventilation and perfusion lung scans (V/Q scan)
  for diagnosis of PE, 166, 168–169, 174–175
Ventricular fibrillation (VF), 58
  amiodarone in, 66–67
  defibrillation of, 58
  lidocaine, 66
Ventricular tachycardia (VT), 210
  defibrillation of, 58
Vessel laceration, 240
VF. *See* Ventricular fibrillation (VF)
Vital signs (VS), 232
V/Q scan. *See* Ventilation and perfusion lung
  scans (V/Q scan)
VT. *See* Ventricular tachycardia (VT)